Future Trends IN AIDS

*The proceedings of a seminar organised by the
Department of Health & Social Security, England
on the 23 March 1987
at the Queen Elizabeth II Conference Centre, London*

LONDON : Her Majesty's Stationery Office.

1532429

ISBN 0 11 321128 7

Contents

Foreword

We have before us one of the most significant and serious epidemics of an infectious disease in this country. Predicting the spread of infection, the development of the disease, and the health-care consequences, is a vital and urgent task. This Seminar was convened to bring together an international group of experts who had engaged this problem, to share views, and to debate the outcome of their research.

The meeting was a great success and those attending agreed to publication of the papers presented, and the questions and discussion that followed. The result is an invaluable review of what we know and what we still need to discover about the future spread of HIV infection and AIDS. It has not been possible of course to check every detail with those who spoke, especially those who failed to give their names for the transcript! Perhaps readers would forgive any errors that may have crept into the account.

Sir Donald Acheson KBE
DM DSc FRCP FFCM FFOM

Opening

The Right Honourable Norman Fowler

Could I say, first, I am very pleased to open this important seminar.

Containing the spread of AIDS is a top priority, not only in this country, but throughout the world. Our strategy has four major parts:

First, public health measures, such as screening of blood donations;

Second, public education so people can learn how to avoid infection;

Third, research into vaccines against HIV infection and treatment for those who are infected;

And fourth, the development of services for those who are infected or have the disease itself.

But to carry forward this strategy, we need to do all we can to obtain the best information. Good planning requires good intelligence. To do this, we need to share our knowledge internationally. No country has a monopoly of wisdom. We must all learn from each other. The gravity of the threat of AIDS reinforces the need for such international cooperation.

I have followed this myself in visits that I have paid to the World Health Organisation, to Berlin, to Amsterdam and to San Francisco, Washington and New York. I learned a great deal from each of those visits, and therefore I am doubly pleased that this is truly an international seminar. I would like to welcome the participants from overseas, particularly those of you who have made very long journeys indeed to come here this morning.

The concern of the Seminar is with future trends in the spread of HIV infection and AIDS. Predictions on these issues are bound to contain great uncertainty and particularly is that so in the longer term, but nevertheless, it is essential that estimates should be made so that our responses can be properly planned. These estimates must try, as far as is possible, to reflect two concerns:

First, they should describe the ranges of possible growth of HIV infection and of AIDS, and

Second, they should recognise that absolute precision is neither possible nor sensible.

So much obviously depends on what individuals do to change their behaviour and the success of researchers in developing vaccines and treatment.

Our predictions must be as soundly based as is possible, but we must be careful that they are not seen as being more precise than they can be.

Our experience in the United Kingdom, at any rate in an international context, is relatively limited and it is therefore important that we learn from other countries. In particular, the numbers here are relatively small and do not provide as reliable a base for predictions as the higher figures in the United States, where AIDS and HIV infection are much more prevalent. There are many lessons, I believe, for us in the American experience.

We do, however, in this country, have an excellent confidential voluntary reporting system for AIDS cases and for results of HIV antibody tests, operated by the Communicable Disease Surveillance Centre of the Public Health Laboratory Service and by the Communicable Disease (Scotland) Unit.

Good reporting systems are essential for good predictions, but no system is flawless. In making our forecasts, we must make proper allowance for that: we should consider how reliable our systems are and whether there are further steps we can take to improve those systems.

It is now time to allow you to proceed with your discussions. I have no doubt that they will help to clarify the understanding of how this disease is likely to develop in the United Kingdom and the steps that we can take to stop it from spreading. No doubt, you will also identify the priorities for further work. This will all be of enormous assistance as far as the Government is concerned and it will also be of great public interest.

It is only by providing professionals and the public with the widest understanding of the issues that we can hope to mobilise their full support and full help in the fight against AIDS.

Ladies and gentlemen, obviously AIDS is a threat to all nations, but in that very threat it has led to a greater building of bridges between nations and I am sure that in working together today we will strengthen those bridges still further.

So I very much look forward to your discussions. I wish you well and I will now hand you back to Donald Acheson.

First Session

Chairman Professor Francis O'Grady
Chief Scientist
Department of Health & Social Security, England

Paper 1

Professor R A Anderson
Imperial College, University of London

Data needs and a theoretical transmission model

Despite remarkable advances over the past 3 to 4 years in our understanding of the basic biology of the human immunodeficiency virus (HIV) at the molecular, cellular and immunological levels, public health planning continues to be hampered by uncertainties about key epidemiological variables. We need to know the typical duration and intensity of infectiousness of HIV seropositives, the fraction that will eventually go on to develop AIDS, and the time-scale of this conversion. Accurate information about HIV seropositives will emerge only from carefully designed studies on time-scales varying in length from many years to many decades. The reason for this is very straightforward:

1. The incubation period of the infection, defined as the time-interval from infection to the diagnosis of disease, is very long. Current estimates would put it in the order of 5 to 8 years and Professor Sir David Cox will be talking about some work at Imperial College, using American data on transfusion-associated cases of AIDS, on the latest estimates of the duration of the incubation period.

2. The full distribution of the incubation period in HIV seropositives will only be known when infected patients have been monitored over a period equivalent to the normal life expectancy of a specified uninfected population matched for age, sex and ethnic (= genetic) background. So under the worst case, that could be many decades before we know the full distribution of the incubation period.

In the absence of such information, mathematical or statistical models of the transmission dynamics of HIV cannot be used at present to make precise quantitative predictions of longterm trends in the incidence of AIDS. They can, however, be used for a variety of purposes and I would like to mention five:

a. to make short-term projections, based on current trends, over 2 to 4 years;

b. to facilitate the indirect assessment of certain key epidemiological parameters;

c. to clarify what data is required to refine predictions;

d. to make predictions under clearly specified assumptions about the course of infection in individuals and about the prevailing patterns of sexual activity in a community;

e. to provide a template to guide the interpretation of observed trends, to facilitate understanding of future trends, and to identify key scientific questions.

In this short talk, I wish to cover four topics very briefly and I am therefore going to exclude technical details which are covered in the references [1,2,3]. The four topics are:

1. What is known about the key epidemiological parameters of HIV transmission;

2. What is not known and needs to be studied;

3. The likely qualitative features of the current epidemic in the United Kingdom;

4. Some future research needs.

If we start by considering what is already known about sexually transmitted diseases, their epidemiologies have been studied for a variety of infections and populations. Some of this knowledge is relevant to the study of the spread of HIV. Firstly, sexually transmitted infections can persist both in low- and high-density populations, unlike many of the common childhood diseases. Secondly, asymptomatic carriers of infection are often important in transmission and this is clearly so for HIV. Thirdly, a degree of immunity does not normally follow recovery from infection. Fourthly, the disease agent often persists in the host for long periods of time and this appears to be true for HIV. Lastly, there is marked heterogeneity of transmission within the population due to great variability in sexual activity in the adult population.

Those are general comments. Now I turn specifically to HIV. The first thing that is known from careful clinical studies of groups of patients is how the trend in the proportion infected in the same population changes through time, and Figure 1 simply illustrates four studies — three in homosexual communities and one in Italy primarily covering drug abuse[1]. In these four studies, the similarities are more important than the differences and the doubling time is of the order of 10 to 12 months throughout Europe and North America.

The doubling time tells about the net transmission of the virus in the community and about the various parameters that determine its magnitude[1]. The doubling time is best derived from serological data rather than changes in incidence of AIDS. Values derived from AIDS case-reports are somewhat unreliable for reasons associated with the long and variable incubation period of the disease and the lag between diagnosis and reporting.

Table 1 provides a summary of various estimates of the doubling time. The similarities are more striking scientifically than the differences given the wide range of sexual activity and of intravenous drug abuse in different communities.

Figure 1

Longitudinal studies of changes in the proportion of cohorts with antibodies to HIV (sources listed in May & Anderson 1987).

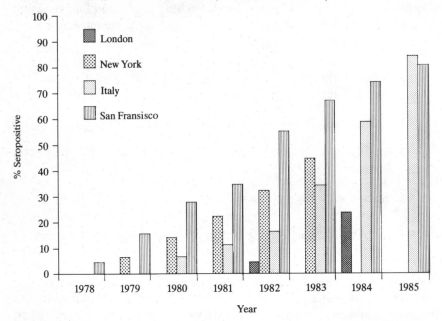

Table 1

Estimates of the doubling time in months of the incidence of cases of AIDS in various localities.

Country	Period	Doubling Time (months)	Rate per year
F.R. Germany	1980–85	8.8	0.94
Australia	1983–85	4.8	1.73
Canada	1981–85	9.3	0.89
Austria	1983–85	15.6	0.53
Spain	1982–85	7.9	1.05
Sweden	1983–85	8.0	1.04
Switzerland	1983–85	9.9	0.84
Italy	1983–85	5.0	1.66
England	1982–85	6.5	1.27
USA	1981–85	9.2	0.90
Average		**8.5**	**1.08**

The topic, which I only want to touch on briefly, is the incubation period of the virus. Figure 2 shows data from Dr Tom Peterman of the Centers for Disease Control from transfusion-associated cases. On the vertical axis is the number of infected cases that developed AIDS and on the horizontal axis is the incubation period in years from infection. There are a number of

Figure 2

The observed distribution of the incubation period of AIDS in patients infected by blood transfusion or blood products (source Dr T Peterman, CDC Atlanta).

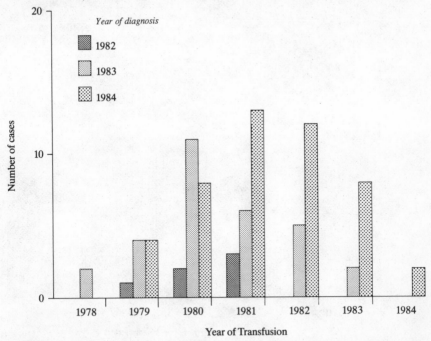

important features reflected in this. You can see that the distribution is highly variable, that it has a long tail and most importantly, that it has a high average value. Clearly, such distributions are truncated, as the length of study of infected patients continues then one expects this distribution to develop a longer tail. Current estimates of the mean incubation period are of the order of 8 years or more[4].

The next question concerns our sexual habits and I would just like to turn to two quantitative studies. The first is by McManus and concerns homosexuals in London[1]. It records one of the most important epidemiological variables in the transmission of the virus, the rate of sexual partner changer per unit of time.

Figure 3 is for a relatively high-risk group, where you can see that there is a high mean and variability in the rate of partner change per year. The mean of this distribution is of the order of 20 to 30 partners per annum but it has an extremely high variance with "professionals" clearly in the tail of the distribution. We need much more hard quantitative data about the pattern of sexual partner change.

If one turns to heterosexuals, how do these distributions look in the heterosexual community in the UK? We have just finished one such study in conjunction with the Harris Research Organisation which I believe is the first quantitative survey in Britain. This was for a relatively small pilot sample of about 800 people and records the average number of partners per year by age-group from those age 18–20 up to the older groups[1].

Figure 3

The frequency distribution of the number of different sexual partners per two-year period in a study of homosexual/bisexual males in London 1984 (data from McManus).

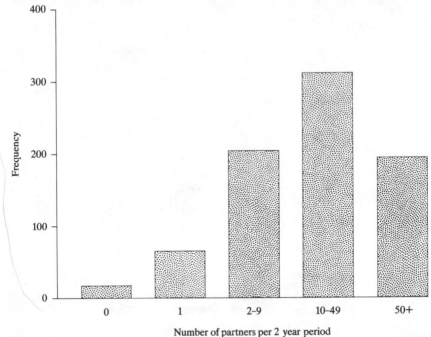

Number of partners per 2 year period

As you can see from Figure 4, this distribution has a very different pattern from that recorded in Figure 3 and the actual overall mean of this distribution is about 1.4, but with a high variance and a long tail. So there could be a difference of the order of 20-fold in the mean rate of sexual partner change between heterosexuals and homosexuals. This does raise an important epidemiological property — namely, in the absence of a high mean for this distribution, is this virus self-sustaining in the heterosexual community? The existence of certain key unknowns, eg the infectiousness of infected patients throughout the incubation period, prevents us from answering this question precisely. The likelihood is however, that it will be self-sustaining. In the early stages of the epidemic cases in heterosexuals are most likely to arise via bisexual men and intravenous drug abusers.

Those are some simple illustrations of what we know quantitatively — not qualitatively — and you might be struck by the relative paucity of that information. Clearly, it is possible to acquire much more information of this type and I rather hope that we can return to this topic later on in this seminar.

The only precise quantitative study of the rate of partner change in relation to the probability of acquiring the disease is by Winkelstein[5] in an unbiased sample of male homosexuals in San Francisco as shown in Figure 5. It shows the percentage of HIV seropositives as a function of the number of male partners per annum, the solid area is the association between the

Figure 4
The frequency distribution of the number of different sexual partners of the opposite sex per one-year period in a study of heterosexuals in England 1986 (May & Anderson 1987).

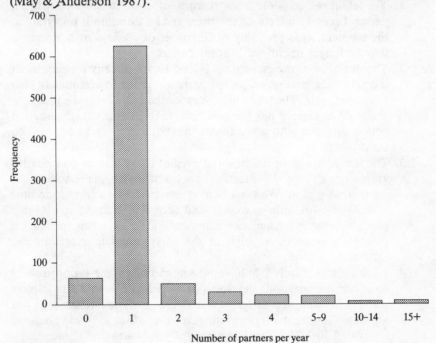

Figure 5
The relationship between sexual activity amongst a sample of homosexual/ bisexual males from San Fransisco USA as measured by the number of different male partners over a two-year period, and the percentage of each group who were seropositive for HIV antibodies (Winkelstein et al 1987).

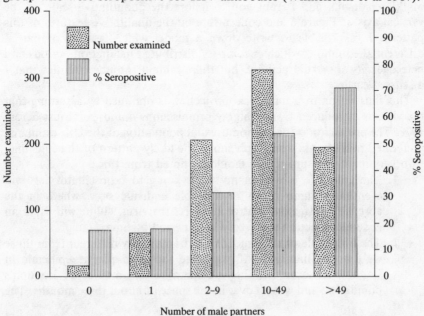

likelihood of seropositivity — in other words infection — and the number of male partners, and this correlation is very high indeed.

If we turn to what is unknown the most important factors are as follows:

1. The latent period is the interval from infection to the point when a person becomes infectious to others and its duration is uncertain at the moment. It is probably of the order of 20 days or more but it may be longer or shorter in some patients.

2. The duration of the incubation period I have already mentioned. It is a very long incubation period so data is going to accumulate on a slow time scale. The transfusion-associated cases form the best data available at present but the need now is to examine the incubation period in those who are infected by sexual activity as opposed to transfusion.

3. The most important unknown at present is the lack of quantitative knowledge of how the infectious period of patients is related to the incubation period. We need hard quantitative data from long time scale studies of viral excretion and secretion because it is highly probably that infectiousness will vary widely over this incubation period. It is probably high in the early and late stages of the incubation period.

4. Equally importantly, we have no knowledge of the proportion of seropositives that will develop AIDS ultimately, and this clearly could differ amongst different at-risk groups. The estimates, as you are all well aware, have been rising, starting off at 15% and going up to around 30%. A recent German study indicates that immunological deterioration occurs over an eight-year period in about 75% of patients. But clearly, it is going to be a long time before one ultimately understands this issue.

Given those uncertainties, it is extremely difficult to provide quantitative predictions but I am now going to talk about the likely qualitative patterns of this epidemic, and I want you to ignore the quantitative scale on the vertical axis of Figure 6 and concentrate on the qualitative features of this pattern. It is possible to write down a model which is a set of partial differential equations which encompass distributed incubation periods and heterogeneity in sexual activity, but there remain the uncertainties that I discussed earlier.

This illustration of a numerical projection is obtained by assuming that the virus is introduced from a highly promiscuous homosexual just before 1978. The projection is for the homosexual population of the UK, estimated at about 2 million, and the graph shows the likely pattern of the epidemic. Two very important properties should be noted from this:

1. The epidemic is not, in my view, going to be oscillatory. It will eventually damp down to a stable endemic state where in the absence of effective control measures the virus will be with us as an endemic infection for a very long period of time.

2. The time scale of this epidemic is dramatically different from those we are familiar with. If you take the 1665 plague epidemic in London for example, this took away about a third of London's population and was all over in the space of about three months. The

Figure 6

The predictions of a hybrid model of the likely qualitative patterns of the AIDS epidemic in the male homosexual community in the UK in the absence of changes in sexual behaviour. The graph records the incidence of AIDS (Anderson et al 1986, 1987).

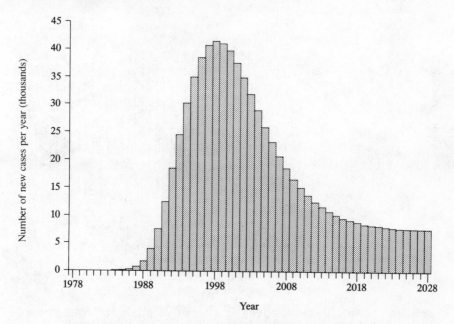

AIDS epidemic, because of its long incubation period, is going to be moving on a time scale of many decades, even in the homosexual community where the rate of partner change is very high.

If I plotted a similar graph for the heterosexual community, given all the uncertainties, one would expect this epidemic to be moving on an even slower time scale over very many decades, and that is an important point to emphasise. Changes here in Britain at the moment could have a dramatic impact on the peak of the epidemic in the future.

If one translates that sort of qualitative picture for AIDS itself into one for HIV seropositivity, Figure 7 shows the equivalent pattern. This gives a rather different picture where in the endemic state in the homosexual community one might end up with a relatively high proportion of infected people. The question mark is whether they will be infectious.

I want to stress that those patterns are critically dependent on prevailing levels of heterogeneity in sexual activity within the UK, and this is well illustrated by Figure 8. We can dissect these figures to ask how quickly will the epidemic move between different sexual partner rate change groups. Supposing I take homosexuals with 1−2 partners per year and then 5−10 partners, 20−50 partners, then 100-plus partners and so on, this is the predicted qualitative pattern and how it will move through these different groups.

In the very high partner-change group, virtually all will be infected, but with lower partner-change groups and particularly the very low one, one

Figure 7
Predictions as in Figure 6 but recording changes in the proportion sero-positive for HIV.

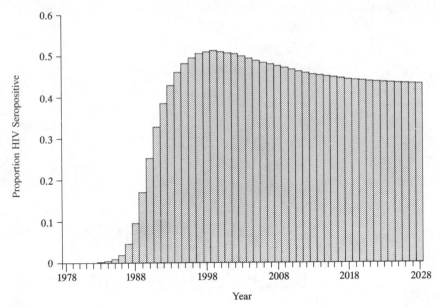

Figure 8
Predicted changes in seropositivity in a series of groups of male homo-sexuals stratified by their rate of sexual partner change (Anderson et al 1986, 1987).

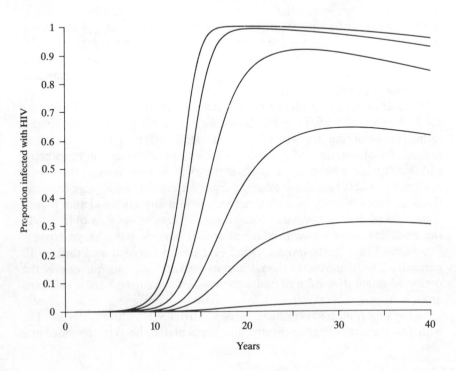

would have very different time scales and patterns of the epidemic. Therefore, it is clear that quantifying sexual activity, as the rate of partner-change, is a very important determinant of the overall pattern. It is the average rate of partner change, weighted by the abundance of each group in the population and the variance within each group, that will determine the overall pattern of the epidemic in the total community.

Figure 9
Prediction of the "minimum size" of the AIDS epidemic in the male homosexual community in the UK under the assumption that all transmission ceased at the end of 1986. The different lines record different assumptions about the proportion of infected individuals who develop AIDS (1.0, 0.8, 0.5 and 0.3). The incubation period was set at 5 years (Anderson et al 1987).

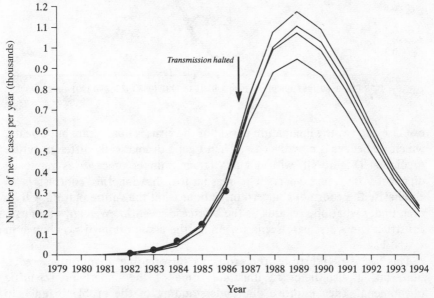

Lastly, I want to turn to the UK situation, in particular the cases amongst the homosexual community, which of course are the dominant number at present. Figure 9 takes these reported cases up to 1986, and shows a fitted model which has a distributed incubation period and heterogeneity in sexual habits as scored by the quantitative data shown earlier. We try to mimic this trend and then take the optimistic assumption that transmission has ceased this year as a result of the educational campaign. I am only doing this as an illustrative point, not that I believe that transmission will cease this year.

The different trajectories beyond 1987 reflect different assumptions about the proportion who will develop AIDS and the length of the incubation period. The highest one is about 70%, the lowest between 15 and 30%, so there will be differences in the pattern and even in transmission and we have a very substantial number of cases as yet to be diagnosed. The graph is for an incubation period of 5 years but supposing I repeat that

Figure 10

Prediction at in Figure 9 but with the average incubation period set at 8 years (Anderson et al 1987).

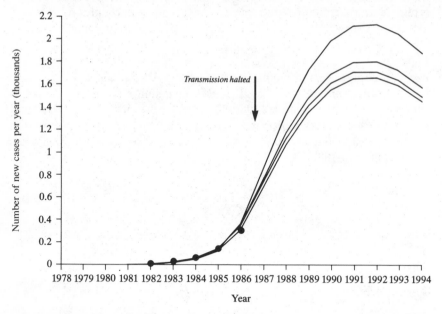

exercise and say the incubation period of the virus is not 5 years but 8 years, which we believe is now the case. Then I get a dramatically different future prediction (Figure 10) with a much larger number of cases as yet to be diagnosed in future years. The reason for showing this contrast is to emphasise the enormous uncertainty about what the future pattern will be even under what one regards as the best case scenario. We can, of course, construct the worst case scenario, under the assumption of no change in sexual habits.

This last issue illustrates the problems surrounding quantitative prediction, but it also helps to illustrate some of the underlying scientific phenomena. They improve our understanding of the problem and help identify the data needs. One has not to be too impatient about these because epidemiological research on a virus with an incubation period of a minimum of 8 years is going to take many decades to clarify the current uncertainties.

One can make predictions about worst and best cases, but beyond that I think it is rather difficult. We need data from quantitative studies of rates of partner change in both heterosexual and homosexual communities. In an ideal world, one would have liked such information before the current educational campaign commenced and one would now like cohort studies of the same groups throughout the impact of the educational campaign, because this rate change is such an important variable in dictating the pattern.

We must have good serological data of AIDS. The interpretation of changes in the incidence is fraught with all sorts of difficulties due to biases in reporting, the lag between diagnosis and reporting, and so on. We need extensive serological studies in this country. Linked to both of these is the reality that precise epidemiological information is going to emerge on a very long time scale and we just have to be patient concerning the rate of acquisition of such knowledge.

References

1. *May RM and Anderson RM*
   The transmission dynamics of HIV infection
   Nature 1987; **326**; 137–142

2. *Anderson RM et al*
   A preliminary study of the transmission dynamics of the human immunodeficiency virus (HIV), the causative agent of AIDS
   IMA J Maths Appl Med Biol 1987; **3**; 229–263

3. *Anderson RM et al*
   Is it possible to predict the minimum size of the acquired immunodeficiency syndrome (AIDS) epidemic in the United Kingdom
   Lancet 1987; **i**; 1073–1075

4. *Winkelstein W et al*
   Sexual practices and risk of infection by the human immunodeficiency virus: the San Francisco men's health study
   JAMA 1987; **257**; 321–325

5. *Medley GF, Anderson RM, Cox DR and Billard L*
   The incubation period of acquired immune deficiency syndrome (AIDS) in patients infected via blood transfusion
   Nature 1987; **328**; 718–721

Questions

Dr JWG Smith
Could I ask how firm the data are relating the proportion of seropositivity to frequency of sexual partner change. One might expect that the ease of transmission would depend not only on the number of partners but also on the type of sexual activity undertaken with, for example, receptive anal intercourse being most important. Also it may depend upon the frequency of sexual activity with each partner during this changing period?

Professor Anderson
This is obviously an important question. There are many complications in interpreting sexual activity data but we have such limited quantitative data that one has to start somewhere. The easiest variable to score is the rate of partner change, and the reason for choosing that variable first is that it is clearly one of the most important determinants if one is concerned with spread through populations. The study of Winkelstein published this year is

the first study in which the group studied was carefully chosen and consisted of homosexuals who were not selected for high risk but were sampled much more randomly than in previous studies. Therefore these are the best quantitative data we have at present. In future there is going to be a series of studies emerging which try to relate the type of sexual activity plus frequency of partner change with levels of seropositivity.

Professor Knox
As well as different types of sexual behaviour and changes of intensity with age, the problem that has been exercising my mind is the idea of a sexual career, because people change their sexual qualitative patterns as well as their quantitative patterns as they age. Obviously when one has even two people who are in the same category at the moment, if they have had different sexual careers up to that point and they have widened their repertoires in different ways, they are going to be quite different from a risk point of view. Trying to represent this either mathematically or on a computer is extraordinarily difficult, I have spent many train journeys so far without success, I wondered if you have tackled this?

Professor Anderson
It again is an important question. The study of heterosexuals in the UK in conjunction with Harris was age and sex stratified. The rate of sexual partner change was age-related and differed between the sexes too. Of course, it is possible to write down sets of equations in which sexual activity is both age and sex dependent. There is no problem in writing down such equations but the reason that one does not at the moment is that we need the data first to facilitate the development of realistic models.

Dr P Mortimer
I was very interested in the point that Roy Anderson raised whether all those who are seropositive are equally infectious. I think we are being very simplistic about this point and I would like to propose that in virological terms it is rather likely that those who have been recently infected are much more infectious than other seropositives because they remain fit and are still sexually active. If that were the case, how does he think it might alter his view of how the epidemic is going to develop?

Professor Anderson
Interesting question. Our initial assumption about change of infectiousness during the incubation period was that it is high in the early stages of infection then drops to a low level because viraemia drops to a low level. There is however limited evidence that virus counts start to rise towards the time when AIDS is diagnosed. Once we have some precise quantitative distribution of that infectiousness, then we can insert it into these models. The important point at the moment is to consider that infected individuals are potentially infectious throughout the incubation period although the distribution will undoubtedly vary through that time.

Sir Donald Acheson

How firm is your estimate of the number of homosexuals. The appropriate figure to use could perhaps be the number of homosexuals who engage in anal intercourse, which probably is a smaller number?

Professor Anderson

The estimate of the number of homosexuals in Britain is pure guesswork at the moment which again comes back to the issue that we urgently need extensive studies of sexual behaviour in the UK. Your second point about particular sexual practices is critically important. I think though, as with the heterosexual community, one is primarily concerned with penetrative sex as a primary risk factor.

Paper 2

Dr Meade Morgan
AIDS Unit
Centers for Disease Control, Atlanta, USA

The empirical prediction model of the Public Health Service

In May 1986, the United States Public Health Service convened a meeting of about 90 scientists in Coolfont West Virginia to help plan the Government's response to the Acquired Immune Deficiency Syndrome (AIDS) crisis[1]. The scientists were divided into groups to address a number of different issues including vaccine development, anti-viral therapies, adequacy of current health-care facilities and other topics. I would like to focus on the work of the demographic projections group. This group was given the responsibility to project both the number of cases that would occur in the United States between 1986 and 1991 as well as the current and future number of persons infected with the human immunodeficiency virus (HIV).

One of the best sources of data we have in the US is our AIDS surveillance system. Since the summer of 1981, when AIDS was first recognised, cases have been reported by physicians to State and local health departments and then to the Centers for Disease Control (CDC). While our surveillance data are excellent for monitoring trends, there are some limitations that should be discussed at the outset. One obvious problem is in the completeness of reporting of AIDS cases to the CDC. The case definition used for AIDS is very restrictive, for a case to be counted, one of about 11 opportunistic diseases must be diagnosed by a method that the CDC considers reliable. Recently we have found that many clinicians who have experience with AIDS are treating patients without the sometimes costly diagnostic procedures that are required under the AIDS definition. Validation studies done in a number of high incidence areas around the US suggest that as many as 10% of diagnosed cases may go unreported[2]. Additional cases may also be occurring that are not recognised as being AIDS. Without scientific studies it is hard to estimate the level of under-recognition, but we speculate that an additional 10% or more of cases are missed. Thus the totals for reported AIDS cases used by CDC are likely 20% too low[1]. Finally, there are other manifestations of HIV infection that our current definition does not include as AIDS. Still, our data for AIDS have been consistently collected over the past six years and provide an excellent way of monitoring the spread of the disease. These data were used at the Coolfont meeting in making our projections through 1991.

Figure 1 illustrates the procedure used. First we counted the number of cases reported to CDC by month of diagnosis. We then adjusted the case

Figure 1

Number of AIDS cases in the United States projected from cases reported up to 30 April 1986.

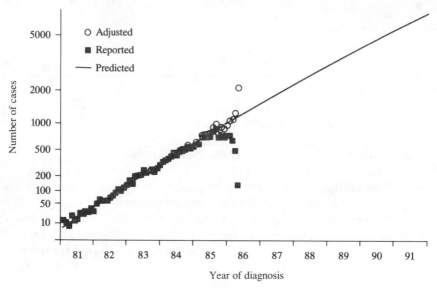

counts for delays which occur in the reporting of cases from physicians to health departments and to CDC. There is on average a 3-month delay between the time a case of AIDS is diagnosed and the time we receive the report. In some instances the delays are large; only 95% of cases are reported within one year of diagnosis. Therefore, even if we look back a year or more, there is still some adjustment that needs to be made. The circles in Figure 1 represent the estimates of the number of AIDS cases diagnosed in each month which will eventually be reported.

The next step was to find a scale that was most suitable for modelling the trends. Because the epidemic appeared to increase exponentially in its early stages, we considered modelling the data by taking the logarithm of the case counts. However the residuals under this approach were ill-behaved. Instead, we used the Box-Cox transformation[3], letting the data suggest which scale was best. The best scale was found to be roughly a cube-root, which the y-axis in Figure 1 reflects. Notice that on this scale a straight line would fit the data pretty well, even though the transformation was not done for that purpose. We considered a series of polynomial models and fit them under the Box-Cox transformation using maximum likelihood techniques. The best fitting polynomial, a quadratic, was used to project incident cases through to 1991.

Figure 2 shows the observed number of diagnosed cases by quarter and the projections after transforming back to the original scale. Confidence bounds of 68% are given rather than the usual 95% because we felt that these would be more meaningful for public health planning. The model indicates that in 1991, 74,000 new cases of AIDS will be diagnosed[4], with bounds ranging from 46,000 to 91,000 cases. That compares with a cumulative total of just over 33,000 cases reported to the CDC up to March

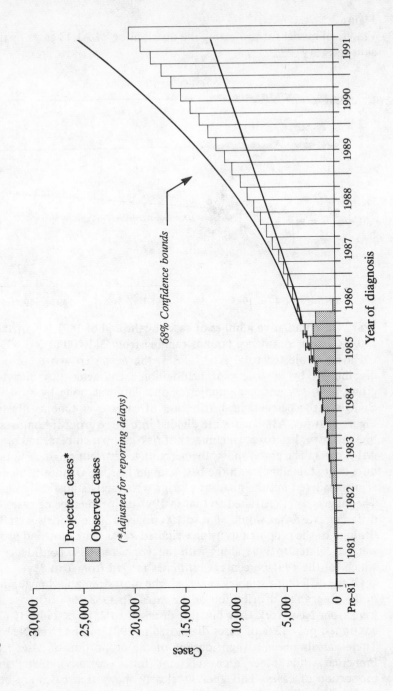

Figure 2
The incidence of AIDS in the United States by quarter of diagnosis. Projected from cases reported up to 30 April 1986.

Meade Morgan

Figure 3
Empirical model for projecting the distribution of AIDS cases by transmission category

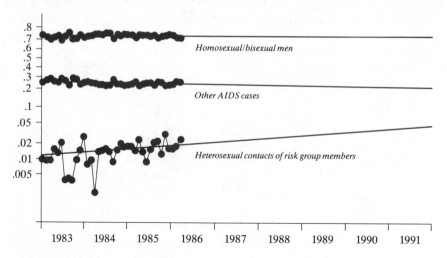

1987. The cumulative number of cases by the end of 1991 is projected to be 270,000, with confidence bounds ranging from 211,000 to 301,000.

Having projected total AIDS cases, the next step was to project their distribution by a variety of demographic characteristics including risk group, age, sex and geographic region. This was done by modelling the change in the percentage distribution of cases over time as illustrated in Figure 3. Adult AIDS cases are divided into three groups: homosexual and bisexual men, heterosexual contacts of risk-group members, and other adult AIDS cases. The graph shows the percentage distribution of cases by month on a logit scale along with the best straight line fit. Quadratic models were also considered but the quadratic terms were rarely statistically significant. The models were restricted so that in 1991 the percentage of cases over the different categories would sum to 100 per cent. The models were fitted to the logit of the proportions using weighted linear regression and projections were calculated to 1991 along with the associated 68% confidence bounds which for the 1991 percentage estimates ranged from 1 to 3%.

Of the different variables analyzed, the most dramatic change was found in the geographic distribution of the cases. In 1983 36% of those reported were from New York City but this declined to 25% in 1986. If the trend continues, only 12% of cases diagnosed in 1991 will be from New York[4]. There has also been a slight decline of the proportion of cases from San Francisco while other areas account for a correspondingly increased proportion of cases. This analysis clearly shows that cases are becoming more widely distributed across the United States. Since the trends we are now seeing in reported cases are lagging many years behind the spread of the virus, the virus is certainly more diffusely spread over the nation than the current case totals would suggest.

There has been only slight change in the distribution of cases by sex. A small increase is projected for the proportion of cases involving adult women who accounted for a total of 6.6% of adult cases reported in 1983. This increased to 7.7% in 1986 and is projected to reach nearly 10% in 1991. The increase in cases among women corresponds to a slight shift in the distribution of patients by transmission category (or risk group). The biggest change we have seen is in the number of cases representing heterosexual transmission from risk group members, the majority of which are women. Only 0.9% of cases diagnosed in 1983 were among the heterosexual contact group, but this increased to 2% in 1986 and is projected to reach 5% of 1991 cases.

Projecting the number of cases was much easier than projecting the number of persons who either were or will be infected with the AIDS virus. We quickly decided not to try to project future infections, concentrating instead on estimating the number currently infected. No population based serologic studies had been done and most seroprevalence data then available was from studies of high risk individuals. The best that could be done was some educated guesswork, illustrated in Table 1. The first step was to estimate the size of the different populations at risk. Using data from Kinsey's 1948 study of sexual behaviour among men[5], roughly 2.5 million men in the United States have been exclusively homosexual throughout their lives and as many as an additional 7.5 million have had some homosexual activity that would put them at risk for infection. The seroprevalence among homosexuals was estimated to range between 10 and 18%, giving somewhere between 690,000 and 1,190,000 homosexual men infected. The

Table 1

Coolfont estimates of HIV prevalence in the United States by population group 1986. Sources: Kinsey et al 1948[1], US Census data 1980[1], National Institute on Drug Abuse[2], National Hemophilia Foundation[3].

Population	Estimated Size	Approximate Seroprevalence	Total Infected
1. Exclusively homosexual throughout life[1]	2,500,000	18%	440,000
2. Other homosexual contact[1]	2,500,000–7,500,000	10%	250,000–750,000
3. Regular (at least weekly) intravenous drug abuse[2]	750,000	30%	225,000
4. Less frequent IV drug use[2]	750,000	10%	75,000
5. Persons with Hemophilia[3]	14,000	70%	10,000
6. Other groups (transfusion recipients, other heterosexuals, infants)	?	?	?
Total			**1,000,000–1,500,000**

process was repeated for intravenous drug users and haemophiliacs. Infections due to heterosexual transmission and transfusion were not included since they likely account for a relatively small number of infections. The estimate for the overall number of infected persons came to between 1.0 and 1.5 million. If correct, the larger figure translates to one infection for every 160 persons in the US population.

Studies have shown that between 20% and 30% of individuals go on to develop AIDS within five years of infection. Thus our projections for future AIDS cases are consistent with the estimate for the number now infected. Nevertheless, I must stress that the models used for projecting are purely empirical and based solely on observed trends in reported AIDS surveillance data. The models serve only as approximations to whatever disease process is generating the data, and will not necessarily hold into the future. The reported confidence bounds should be considered an overestimate of our true confidence. Nevertheless, the empirical models do, at least for the short to middle term, give us some numbers to use in developing public health policy. They have been very useful in seeing that proper funds go into research and in helping us prepare to meet the health care needs of those who are expected to develop AIDS in the near future.

References

1. *Coolfont Report*
   A PHS plan for the prevention and control of AIDS and the AIDS virus
   Public Health Reports 1986; **101**; 341–348

2. *Hardy AM et al*
   Assessing the level of AIDS case-reporting by review of death certificates
   Public Health Reports 1987; (in press)

3. *Box GEP and Cox DR*
   An analysis of transformations
   J Royal Statistical Soc (series B) 1964; **26**; 211–252

4. *Morgan WM and Curran JW*
   Acquired immunodeficiency syndrome: current and future trends
   Public Health Reports 1986; **101**; 459–465

5. *Kinsey AC, Pomeroy WB and Martin CE*
   Sexual behaviour in the human male
   Philadelphia 1948: WB Saunders

Questions

Professor Anderson
I would very much agree with your comment that these sorts of empirical models are good over one to two years but thereafter they have extremely wide bounds. I was interested in how you feel about heterosexual spread. If

you take the rise in the doubling time in heterosexuals it is much the same as in the homosexuals and even a bit faster at present. At the beginning, the change will be pumped by the bisexual IV drug abusers and therefore the early stages are totally misleading about what is going to happen later. The impression is that there is a much lower rate of partner change, so after an initial period of pumping, the doubling time will then lengthen dramatically in the heterosexual community. Do you believe that?

Dr Meade Morgan

I would agree with you on that. There are several other problems in the data also. There might be a reporting bias when people are reporting risk factor information with a tendency to lie about the type of sexual encounter. I would feel it easier to say that I had gone to bed with a prostitute than with the man next door, so we feel that there might be a reporting bias in terms of the apparent increase in the number of heterosexual cases. That is certainly true.

Dr Reid

Professor Knox mentioned the sexual careers. Could I ask about the reporting record of clinicians with longer experience in the USA. We are certainly aware of some reluctance to label a person with AIDS, say on a death certificate for example, and of course this is a variable which hopefully will improve. Has this happened in the USA?

Dr Meade Morgan

We do know of some instances where it has happened. We feel, in talking with the physicians that see the majority of the AIDS patients around the country, that it is not a very big problem but we do not have any hard data to make any estimates of under-reporting.

Paper 3

Professor Klaus Dietz
Tübingen University

Models of transmission in a heterosexual population

I feel honoured to be able to address this distinguished audience and to contribute to the important discussion on the analysis of future trends on AIDS.

So far mathematicians and epidemiologists who were involved in the development of models for infectious diseases, usually had at their disposal data after an epidemic or equilibrium data to which an existing or newly developed model could be fitted. Here, we are in a completely new situation, a new agent has entered the population and we have heard in the previous talk by Professor Anderson that even basic characteristics like the duration of the infectious period or the degree of infectiousness are not known, let alone the contact parameters. Therefore, quantitative work in this context offers great difficulty. There are certain basic features of epidemic theory, however, which are extremely important like the identification of thresholds that have to be exceeded for an endemic level to persist. In the classical theory the basic reproduction rate, ie the number of secondary cases, is the product of three quantities: the number of contacts per unit of time, the probability that a contact is infectious if it takes place between a susceptible and an infective, and the average duration of the infectious period.

But with sexually transmitted diseases, this concept can no longer be true because the probability that a partner is infected depends on the duration of a partnership. There have been some attempts to make the probability of infection explicitly dependent on the duration of a partnership. What seems to me important is the truly dynamic consideration of that situation: one would like to use these models to understand what is the minimum number of partners to maintain this infection in the heterosexual population.

Table 1 shows a survey on sexual behaviour in the Federal Republic of Germany which tries to estimate the number of past sexual relationships in a representative heterosexual population of about 600 males and nearly 500 females. You see that the average number of partners so far reported was 6 for the males and about 3 for the females with large standard deviations. Table 2 gives the proportions of individuals who state that the present partnership is longer than a certain limit, so for instance, more than 50% of the individuals give the length of partnership as 8 to 12 years. Table 3 shows the answers to a question on the existence of a partnership at a given point in time. 90% of both males and females report a steady partnership. About

Table 1

Responses about the number of previous sexual relationships in the Sexual Education And Therapy project (SEAT).

	Males(%)	Females(%)
none or no reply	29.8	45.7
one	7.4	11.6
2	7.9	10.2
3 to 5	21.3	18.9
6 to 10	14.6	8.9
11 to 20	11.4	2.7
more than 20	7.6	1.9
	100 (n = 595)	100 (n = 481)
Average number of partners	$\bar{x} = 6.2$	$\bar{x} = 2.8$
	$s = 8.2$	$s = 5.0$

Table 2

Responses about the duration of the present partnership in the SEAT project (cumulative percentages among those who answered).

more than	Males(%)	Females(%)
6 months	87.9	92.6
2 years	81.7	85.2
4 years	73.1	76.5
6 years	64.5	67.8
8 years	59.7	58.7
12 years	45.0	43.4
20 years	22.1	15.1

Table 3

Other responses about the present partnership in the SEAT project.

	Males(%)	Females(%)
At present there is a steady partnership	90.9	90.4
At present there is no steady partnership	7.6	8.7
So far no sexual relationship	1.5	0.8
	100 (n = 595)	100 (n = 481)

sexual relationships outside a present partnership, more than 80% of males and females say that they have no other sexual relationships.

This means that one cannot use these classical approaches which implicitly assume that all contacts within a partnership take place at one point in time after which a partner is immediately available for new partnerships. In the following I will present some results on a model that is very simple but has the advantage that one can explicitly analyse the whole structure of the model with 5 parameters. We assume that an individual enters the population as susceptible which means that vertical transmission (perinatal infection) is neglected. Then at some point, infection takes place and the infection stays with the individual throughout his life.

In order to take into account formation of partnerships, it is assumed that individuals enter the population as single males or single females and then partnerships are formed at a certain rate. A partnership may be terminated for two reasons: death of one partner or by separation of the two partners.

I assume for simplicity that everybody goes back to the sexually active state. You will see that the partnerships now have to be distinguished according to the infective status of the partners. So you have partnerships where both male and female are negative, where the female is positive and the male is negative, the other way round, and where both sexes are positive. Obviously, if there were no contact outside a partnership of two negatives by either partner, then there would be no transition between these types of partnership and one could, mathematically speaking, consider each pair of partners temporarily immune as long as they stay within the partnership. But obviously, as soon as contacts outside the partnership take place, say with an infected prostitute, then an infection may occur.

On the basis of this model, we have an estimate of the minimum number of lifetime partners needed for the persistence of the endemic equilibrium if it is assumed that the infectious period lasts on average 10 years. This is shown in Figure 1 for various probabilities that one sexual contact in the heterosexual population between a susceptible and an infective partner leads to infection. There have been some studies on this parameter where partners of haemophiliacs were followed over several years and it seems that the probability of transfer of infection is very low. There are some estimates which are only of the order of 1 in 2000. That would even be lower than the lowest that is considered in this figure which is 1 in 100.

The duration of a partnership is on a logarithmic scale starting with a few days up to 50 years. On the ordinate, we have the number of partners during lifetime which is also on a logarithmic scale that varies over several orders of magnitude. If the average duration of partnerships is assumed to be small, then one can use the classical model so that the critical number of partners needed is inversely proportional to the infection probability. This means that the classical model would overestimate the critical number of partners needed. If however one takes into account the duration of the partnership, and for instance assumes that it averages one year, then the minimum number of partners during lifetime is considerably reduced and is between 6 and 12 if the infection probability per contact varies between 0.1 and 0.01.

Figure 1

The minimum number of partners needed to sustain the infection in a heterosexual population by duration of partnership. The lines represent varying probabilities (from 0.01 to 0.1) that a single sexual contact between a susceptible and infectious partner will lead to infection. The duration of the infectious period is assumed to be 10 years.

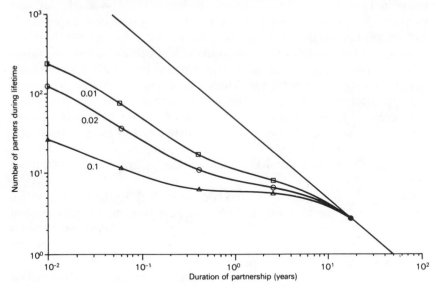

And as the average duration of a partnership increases even further, the critical number declines as well.

Control has quite intricate implications. It is not just sufficient to say it is important to reduce the number of partners during lifetime. One has to specify also how it is done. If one keeps the average duration of the partnerships constant, this moves straight into the area where no endemic equilibrium is possible. If one increases the duration of a partnership, then it could well be that the same reduction in the number of partners during lifetime will not lead to an elimination of the infection.

In terms of dynamic behaviour, it is also quite important to take into account the duration of partnerships because the rate of approach to equilibrium is then reduced, as one would expect because a partnership first has to be terminated before a new contact can take place. Thus, depending on the average number of partners during lifetime, the time of approach to equilibrium can be very long and may take decades.

This is a very simple model. It has the advantage that it can lead to an explicit calculation of all the critical parameters and give some quantitative guidelines but it is obvious that the reality is much more complicated. Certain factors have already been discussed, like age dependence. For instance, there is a strong correlation between the ages of partners, but in addition there is also strong time dependence overall. So the next step would really be to make this model age-dependent. One can expect that the critical number of partners needed for the persistence of the endemic will then increase because a large proportion of the couplings will then be between partners of similar age. As susceptibles enter the sexually active age-groups, the probability that both partners are susceptible will be higher than if there were random mixing irrespective of age.

A second factor which will also need to be included has already been mentioned by Roy Anderson and is the heterogeneity in the present model. It was initially assumed that the parameters are constant for everybody, in reality one has to assume a distribution which has to be taken into account. Lastly, a major methodological point: it is very important to fit these models to the data on HIV and AIDS with any necessary modification obvious from their biology. One can also fit these models to hepatitis B and other sexually transmitted diseases, and these then can help to test these models. I come back to the remark that Roy Anderson made: one needs data first, and then models. In certain cases we already have the data, and we can start building these models.

Reference

1. *Dietz K and Hadeler KP*
   Epidemiological models for sexually transmitted diseases
   Journal of Mathematical Biology; (in press)

Questions

Dr Tyrrell

I understand that in physics and in epidemiology the behaviour of a model can be very much affected by a rather small subset of data. For instance, have you looked at the possibility that changes in the average behaviour of a population, whilst leaving a small subset still with many partners, would alter the predictions you make?

Professor Dietz

Yes, this is known from other fields where one has looked at heterogeneous contact patterns. For instance in my experience with modelling malaria, a small subset of the population that does not take part in chemotherapy can lead to completely different conclusions and can maintain the infection in the whole population. Whilst it is true that the critical parameter, which is usually called the basic reproduction rate, may be greater on average and a smaller contact rate can be sufficient to maintain the infection, yet the overall prevalence is smaller for heterogeneity.

Paper 4

Professor H W Hethcote
University of Iowa, USA

Other modelling work in the USA

I want to describe some models that are being developed at the University of Iowa that are more comprehensive than those that have been presented so far.

Professor Dietz has shown us models that are primarily oriented to a heterosexual population and Professor Anderson has emphasised models that are primarily for a homosexual population. I want to look at models that include both of these and the models will include all of the known HIV transmission mechanisms, including homosexual and heterosexual intercourse, needle sharing among drug abusers, blood transfusions, administration of blood-factor concentrates to haemophiliacs, and perinatal infections where children are infected by their mothers.

The models will also include the known risk groups: the primary risk groups are sexually active homosexual and bisexual men, prostitutes, sexually active heterosexual women and men, drug-abusing women and men. These are called "primary" because there is transmission in both directions, as we will see soon on a compartmental diagram. Secondary risk groups are those who are getting the infection from the primary risk groups, but are not spreading it back to primary risk groups. These include:

1. transfusion recipients and haemophiliacs;

2. monogamous men who have homosexual intercourse with one man in a primary group, for example, homosexual or bisexual men;

3. monogamous women who have heterosexual intercourse with one man in the previous group;

4. monogamous men who have intercourse with one woman in a previous group and children born to women in a previous group.

These groups are related in an interaction diagram, as shown in Figure 1. You can see the primary groups with bidirectional spread between them, for example, homosexual and bisexual men, bisexual men and heterosexual women, heterosexual men and heterosexual woman interacting. The interactions are shown. Notice the unidirectional spread outward, for example, from a heterosexual woman to a monogamous man who has contact with only one woman. The flow in and out of these various groups

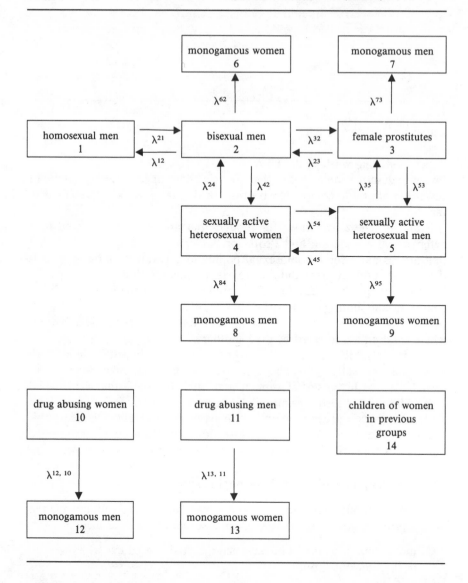

is not shown. There may be a 5–10% movement in and out. Some may cease homosexual activity, some women may become prostitutes and other women may cease being prostitutes.

These primary groups should be divided into subgroups by level of sexual activity. We may need less active, active and more active subdivisions within these groups. This was certainly important in the study of gonorrhoea transmission. Not shown in Figure 1 are compartments for transfusion-recipient children, men and women, nor compartments for haemophiliac boys and men, or for their monogamous partners.

I agree with all of the previous speakers in that parameter estimation is very difficult, particularly in a comprehensive model of this type. However, you can estimate some sexual contact rates by frequencies of interaction, for example, between heterosexual men and prostitutes, between heterosexual men and heterosexual women, and so on. You can estimate transmission probabilities and these are lower from women to men than from men to women. Some would say that a comprehensive model of this type is not possible at this point — it is difficult because of the bounds in estimating parameters. Some estimates can be made and it is important to look at everything together, because you can discover things from a model of this type that you cannot discover by studying, for example, homosexuals only.

You may want to consider the relative importance of sexual transmission and needle sharing transmission. To study needle-sharing transmission, you need to decide on needle-sharing activity levels for the various groups. These are for women and men who are drug-abusing but not in one of the other categories, so they would have a certain activity level in terms of how often they shared needles. Homosexual and bisexual men would have a needle-sharing activity level, also prostitutes and at lower levels, heterosexual women and men. Then, a proportionate mixing approach can be used with those needle-sharing activity levels to come up with a needle-sharing contact matrix.

Perinatal infection can be handled by estimates of birth rates in these primary groups and then, together with the probability of infection and prevalence levels in the various groups, you can estimate the number of children who are infected from their mothers. Simulations can incorporate transmission parameters which change with time. For example, we know that we now have very little, if any, transmission through blood transfusions because of the testing that is now done, very little transmission through blood factor concentrates for haemophiliacs, so the model would have to incorporate that decreased change in transmission to those groups.

Based on a self-reporting and decreased incidence of anorectal gonorrhoea, it is clear that changes in the homosexual behaviour in the US have occurred. Thus in the homosexual population the transmission rate has gone down as a function of time.

So far, the model includes only HIV infection. We need to include AIDS incidence. There are a variety of classification systems. For example there is one that was developed at Walter Reed Hospital by Redfield and others where individuals start out with positive antibody tests, moving on to lymphadenopathy, depletion of T-helper cells, delayed hypersensitivity, thrush and the last category is opportunistic infection. It seems that people do move through a sequence of stages.

Another classification system that has developed for this and other purposes by the Centers for Disease Control has people starting out in acute infection when they first get the HIV infection. That ceases as they move into an asymptomatic phase, after which there is lymphadenopathy and then on into other disease, typified by constitutional disease with fever and weight loss, neurologic diseases such as dementia or neuropathy, and secondary infectious disease such as Pneumocystis carinii. There are also others such as thrush, tuberculosis, secondary cancers, Kaposi's sarcoma, lymphoma. So the point is that individuals seem to move through a sequence of steps towards AIDS and so the model that I propose handles this by placing individuals in the risk groups subdivided by susceptibility. When they become infected, a certain fraction may move into the group that eventually is progressing towards AIDS and another fraction may be infectious but not progressing towards AIDS as shown in Figure 2.

Figure 2
A classification of outcome for susceptible individuals after infection with HIV.

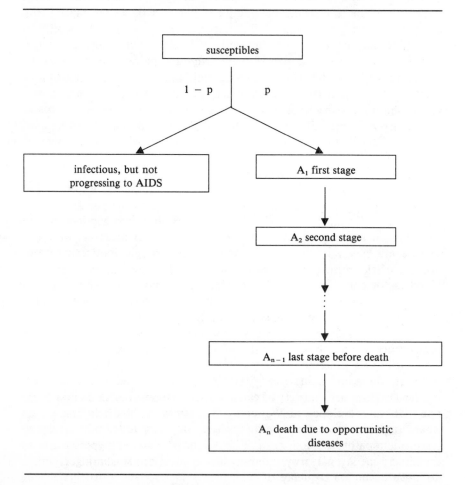

The subdivisions here may depend on the size or the titre of the virus in the initial inoculum. It may depend on the response of the individual at the time of infection. It is possible that $p = 1$ and everybody moves into a stage in which they are infectious and there could be a cofactor that occurs at some time after the initial infection. It has been suggested that this cofactor could be any secondary infection or infection with a lymphotropic virus or something of that particular type.

First Session

Figure 3
Differential equations describing the incidence rates forming the basic model (see text).

$$\frac{d(N_iI_i)}{dt} = (1-p)\sum_{j=1}^{13}(\lambda_{ij}q_j + \eta_{ij})N_j\left(I_j + \sum_{m=1}^{Q}A_{jQ}\right)(1-I_i)$$

$$\frac{d(N_iA_{i1})}{dt} = p\sum_{j=1}^{13}(\lambda_{ij}q_j + \eta_{ij})N_j\left(I_j + \sum_{m=1}^{Q}A_{jQ}\right)(1-I_i) - \gamma_{i1}N_iA_{i1}$$

$$\frac{d(N_iA_{i2})}{dt} = \gamma_{i1}N_iA_{i1} - \gamma_{i2}N_iA_{i2}$$

$$\vdots$$

$$\frac{d(N_iA_{im})}{dt} = \gamma_{im-1}N_iA_{im-1} - \gamma_{im}N_iA_{im}$$

$$\vdots$$

$$\frac{d(N_iA_{in})}{dt} = \gamma_{in-1}N_iA_{in-1}$$

$$\frac{d(N_{14}I_{14})}{dt} = (1-p)b\,\frac{\sum_{women} N_i(I_i + A_{i1} + \cdots + A_{iQ})}{\sum_{women} N_i}$$

$$\frac{d(N_{14}A_{14,1})}{dt} = pb\,\frac{\sum_{women} N_i(I_i + A_{i1} + \cdots + A_{iQ})}{\sum_{women} N_i} - \gamma_{14}N_{14}A_{14,1}$$

$$\vdots$$

$$\frac{d(N_{14}A_{14,m})}{dt} = \gamma_{14,m-1}N_{14,m-1}A_{14,m-1} - \gamma_{14,m}N_{14}A_{14,m}$$

This model is flexible in that it allows a variety of different theories that can be tested. Some data are available on the incubation period and estimates have been made for the mean of that incubation period. Another estimate will be given later on today.

The basic model consists of ordinary differential equations where the incidence rates are governed by usual mass action as shown in Figure 3. So for example, in this model we have 13 major groups that were shown and we have interaction rates that are due to sexual transmission, probability of transmission during a new sexual encounter or in needle-sharing. Some of the people that become infected move into a category and move through the various stages in the progression towards AIDS. The last equations describe the perinatal transmission of mothers to their children.

The uses of a model of this particular type are many, but in particular let me describe these three:

1. You can do a sensitivity analysis to determine the effects of changes in parameters by running the computer simulation model with a range of parameter values and you can detect how that changes the output, the

predictions of the models and indeed determine which parameters are most influential in governing the predictions. Once those are determined, then future studies may be possible in order to get better estimates of those parameters.

2. A use that I think is quite important is to test various prevention approaches. The model is developed, then you can find the effects of an education programme which, for example, leads to consistent condom use by 50% of the heterosexuals. Or we can find out what happens if 80% of the homosexuals practice safe sex; what happens is there is a reduction in needle sharing by 70%; or the effects of vaccinating various fractions of each risk group using vaccine, should one become available. You can answer questions such as how important is needle sharing versus sexual transmission, how important are risk groups — bisexuals, prostitutes etc — in the transmission process.

3. Lastly, I have listed prediction. This is often difficult. You can predict under various assumptions or look at various scenarios and what will happen every month for five to ten years using the computer simulation model, but again, the quality of the predictions will depend on the quality of the data that you used in estimating the model parameters.

So, in conclusion, the model that is being developed is a comprehensive model which considers all risk groups and all known transmission mechanisms up to this time. The benefit of a comprehensive model of this type is that you can use it not only as an experimental tool but also to predict what would happen under various possible changes in sexual and needle-sharing behaviour.

Questions

Professor Anderson
You called this a comprehensive model, and yet it ignores factors such as distributed incubation period and heterogeneity in sexual activity, and I think one has to be very careful in this particular field. It is easy to construct sets of differential equations of arbitrary complexity, arbitrary numbers of parameters but our primary aim initially should be to understand and stimulate the collection of the right sort of data. So on that line, I would like to ask what you have learned epidemiologically from constructing this sort of model?

Professor Hethcote
Well at this point I would say the models are being developed and we have not formulated estimates of all of the parameter values that are needed. The process of formulating models can be very useful to epidemiologists and others, because they must specify precisely what the assumptions are at any given time. It is a useful challenge to the epidemiologist, to provide the answers that are necessary in order to formulate the models.

In response to the other part of your question, the model does include various categories for the several stages in the development of AIDS, and so that can allow a distribution of incubation periods as in some of the other models. I agree with Professor Anderson that it is easy to formulate models of arbitrary complexity and many parameters. I think that one of the dangers of a model of this particular type is inappropriate or unthinking use — so one has indeed to be very careful. I would visualise that the various parts could be isolated and analysed separately, you could analyse the homosexual population first and then move up and add bisexual, prostitutes, heterosexuals later.

The advantage of a comprehensive model is that you have to be consistent with all of the data that have been obtained, so once you obtain the parameter estimates your predictions in various groups have to be consistent with what has been obtained so far. If they are not, then you realise that some of the parameter estimates that you thought were appropriate when you analysed the homosexual population only, may not be that important.

Sir Donald Acheson
I was interested to hear you say that you thought the probability of transmission from an infected male to an uninfected female was possibly greater than in the reverse direction. What evidence exists for this view?

Professor Hethcote
I think some data on that has been collected by the Centers for Disease Control in Atlanta. It is certainly true for gonorrhoea for which available data show that the probability of transmission is higher from an infected male to a susceptible female than from an infected female to a susceptible male. My view is based on the analogy with gonorrhoea and other sexually-transmitted diseases and also on data that have been collected at CDC.

Sir Donald Acheson
If I could comment, it seems certain that the risk is greater for the receiving homosexual than the penetrating homosexual. Whether that has any relevance to the male/female situation I am not sure, but it might.

Dr Peterman
We have limited information on this. We have studied the spouses of transfusion recipients and found of the husbands of women who are infected by transfusions, 2 out of 25 became infected, about 8%. When looking at the wives of infected male transfusion recipients, we found that 10 out of 55 were infected, about 18% — a higher percentage, but not a statistically significant difference.

With regard to gonorrhoea transmission, the studies that have shown differences in rates have really been of different design and are not entirely comparable. Many really believe there is a difference in male to female transmission and the studies that have been done do support a difference but only weakly.

General discussion

Dr McClelland

I think I am right in understanding that the models that have been presented all make an assumption that the risk of heterosexual transmission is constant over the duration of a given partnership. That seems to me to be biologically highly unlikely and I suspect it is more likely to emerge that there will be a population who are efficient transmitters and another population who are not. Could I ask any of the modellers if they could tell us what effect that would have, particularly on the very interesting effects of a longer duration partnership but with a smaller number of partners, as Professor Dietz mentioned?

Professor Anderson

There are so many biological unknowns that my own view on the role of models is that the predictive statistical model over 1 to 2 years is the best we can do at present. The role of formulating models is to focus attention on the acquisition of quantitative data. That is the primary scientific role but linked with exploration of different sorts of biological assumptions one can pose "what if?" questions, the usual scientific procedure to generate understanding.

To give one very simple example, if we take the heterogeneity of sexual activity, a very trivial and simple model can show that this by itself can explain a linear rise in seropositivity through time and can also explain, in a qualitative scientific understanding sense, just how important is the tail of the distribution of sexual activity. It is important as a function of the square of the ratio of the variance to the mean rather than just the mean rate of partner change. Those are sort of qualitative scientific understandings, and my own view is that this is the primary role at present.

Dr Joan Aron

I have a question that relates to what Professor Anderson and Professor Dietz talked about. We are in the business of looking not just at the AIDS end point but at intermediate stages as well.

For infection, you have emphasised strongly that we need more data on the serological aspects of this disease. I agree that would be nice but I am concerned that it is difficult to obtain AIDS reporting that is population-based, at least that is the US experience. There are tremendous difficulties about population-based seroprevalence surveys because they raise the whole issue of identifying people who are infected but not yet ill. It is difficult enough with AIDS but with serology there are likely to be heavy biases. Therefore, should we be putting that much emphasis on it?

On the intermediate stages between infection and AIDS diagnosis, clearly as information becomes available on these stages we can fit the models. I wonder how sensitive is the assumption that there is a predetermined split into those who will progress to AIDS and those who will not. The alternative is to assume at every stage that some people may progress further, some remain in that stage, and possibly that some may even regress. How sensitive are the estimates to variable progression syndromes?

Professor Anderson

I am neither qualified nor competent to comment on the ethical issues about serological sampling, but may I make one simple statement as an epidemiologist who is interested in more precise information. There are a large number of serum banks available in this country, for example my own research group contacted one recently on measles and rubella antibody assessment, and it would in principle be possible to assess on age and sex stratified bands the HIV antibody seroprevalence. The broader ethical reasons I really leave to my medical colleagues.

Professor A Glynn

I would like to take up the point of the relative emphasis we should put on looking at how AIDS data might be helpful in developing a model. It is essentially telling us the history of the infection some five years ago whereas the serological data is telling us what has happened within the last year, and that is really what we would like to know particularly as the scene is changing all the time. Although it may be more difficult to develop antibody data, I suspect in fact we can obtain a far larger number, which makes the mathematics easier. Although ethics are a very difficult problem, my own feeling is that there are not insuperable ethical difficulties about collecting adequate amounts of serological data.

Dr Meade Morgan

We have considered the possibility of trying to devise a population-based sample of the entire US in an attempt to get baseline data on seroprevalence. Then we would repeat this at intervals to look for incidence data or a change in prevalence. There are many methodological problems we would have to face. One of the primary groups that interest us, drug abusers, is going to be hard to find and hard to enroll in the study.

Another of the groups, homosexual men, might decline to participate once they find out what the study is about, so we will have to devise some indirect measures to show prevalence. There are several that are being used in the United States and I think some of them have their counterparts in the United Kingdom. One would be looking at the Red Cross blood screening data for a change in prevalence over time to try and track the spread of the infection. We also have data from all new applicants to the US military forces and from 14 months of data we have seen no increase in prevalence, but there are some reporting biases in that sample, like all others.

One approach that we have just started in a number of hospitals around the country is anonymous screening of all acute admissions that are not related to HIV infection. These data are now becoming available and we will also be looking to them to monitor trends. So I do think that the seroprevalence state is important in formulating models and we need to figure out some way of being able to get data to be able to apply the models that are being proposed.

Professor Adler

Can I pick up that point. If we are going to do national seroprevalence studies, do we necessarily need to get consent? That is where the biases begin to creep in. If the sample is truly anonymous and correctly identified, with on-going sentinel centres that take different cuts of the population and of different medical care agencies, then we should be able to get over those biases. Once we build in a consent, we do create for ourselves quite a problem with potential bias.

Professor Hethcote

I would like to respond to one of the questions that Dr Joan Aron raised. She asked about sensitivity of the results to the split of individuals at the time of infection. At this point I do not know how sensitive they are to that particular split, but that is one of the advantages of the computer simulation models — that you can test various probabilities in various situations to determine how influenced the results are by a particular parameter.

Dr Tyrrell

Years ago when working on respiratory infections, we had similar problems trying to get reasonable figures for infectiousness and transmission rates. We tried to find substitutes for the epidemiological observations we really needed and we included in these estimates the amount of virus present in respiratory secretions, estimates of the infectious dose, plus some estimates of the probability that people who coughed would produce enough virus for somebody adjacent to them to inhale. I wonder whether something comparable to this might be done. It is not an easy option, but it is such a difficult estimate to make by epidemiological methods that it might be worthwhile to try an alternative approach. We would feel very reassured if they both gave roughly the same answer.

Therefore before we leave this question of modelling. I wonder whether anybody has a suggestion for "biological methods" of trying to get at these essential parameters. Would it be worth looking for the amount of virus in semen or cervical secretions, or the number of cells, and then linking that with frequency and style of intercourse to get measures of the likelihood of transmission.

Professor Anderson

I very much agree. What we need initially, and this must be started very quickly, is a longitudinal study of infected patients. The only variable that we can simply score to start with would be something like viral excretion, secretion, or abundance in products. But then again, one has to set up such a study to cover a wide range of different individuals — those who receive infection via sexual transmission, in addition to those who are transfused. Because of the long and variable incubation period, I suspect that there will be a great deal of variability in viral abundance in these different patients. This is not easy, so these studies need to be set up soon and they need to run over long time periods.

In the interim, we can obtain a crude average from the doubling of time of the epidemic. If we know something about the rate and duration of partner change, then we can extract an overall average. At present that is the best we can do.

Professor Adler

The converse to David Tyrrell's comment is that we cannot assume that people are equally susceptible to being infected.

Professor Healy

Could I ask Professor Dietz a question about the definitions of partner change? Taking what must be a common case of a monogamous married man who resorts to many prostitutes on a constant basis, he has one regular partner and a large number of very short-term partners. Is that covered by the models we are talking about?

Professor Dietz

Yes, in the model that I presented, the line for the critical number of partners did not include short-term contacts with prostitutes but I am working on a more extended model which includes these extra contacts either during a partnership or between partnerships.

Dr McClelland

May I make a very brief comment on seroprevalence studies. I welcome what Professor Adler said, but we must not underestimate the enormous difficulties. I speak from personal experience having been trying for months to negotiate an uncoupled seroprevalence study in antenatal patients in the Lothian area of Scotland where this is a highly relevant question to be investigated. It has proved quite unbelievably difficult.

Professor Healy

I am very concerned about a point that both Sir Donald Acheson and Roy Anderson raised, the bridging group and denominators. Presumably, we do now know accurately what the denominator is for homosexual or bisexual men. The assumption that it is 10% is always taken from samples of those attending clinics. We may have a better idea about intravenous drug addicts, but it seeem that our national study of sexual behaviour would need a very large sample because the denominator is going to be reasonably small.

Also, do we believe that bisexual men behave in the same way with their homosexual partners as they do with their heterosexual partners, which must be very important in terms of how quickly infection will get from this bridging group to the heterosexual population. If they behave in the same way heterosexually as they do homosexually, the chances of infecting the heterosexual population must be substantially greater.

Professor Anderson

In support of Michael Healy's comment, it really is so urgent to carry out some national quantitative study of sexual habits, on the bisexual, homosexual and the heterosexual. Some of the present surveys have little value scientifically. It is useless to pose a question by a Gallup Poll which asks: "As a response to the Government's education campaign, have your sexual habits changed? Tick the box YES or NO".

We need a carefully designed study which has questions of a precise quantitative character. Clearly, the information is going to be unreliable in certain areas, but we must do as well as we can to start with and it needs to be done now.

——————————————— End of First Session ———————————————

Second Session

Chairman Dr J W G Smith
Director of the Service
Public Health Laboratory Service, England & Wales

Paper 5

Professor E G Knox
University of Birmingham, England

Predicting the size of the epidemic
I think everybody understands from the modelling representations we have
heard so far that the general principle adopted is to look at a very
complicated situation and begin to simplify it somehow. You either collapse
it down by just looking at the heterosexuals or you collapse it down by not
looking at temporal change or by not looking at age-dependency. No doubt
in the long term, the various modelling approaches will converge upon each
other but for the moment we are all having to simplify quite considerably
and my model is just another example within that theme[1].

My simplification was to get rid of time and see if we could predict what
equilibrium state would be reached eventually without having to consider
the rate of approach towards that equilibrium. I thought the best method of
presentation might be to start with an example of the results of the
calculation, in a graphic format, then work back to the questions and to the
methods which produced these results.

Figure 1
The equilibrium AIDS profile of partner change-rates and HIV prevalences by behavioural
group. For symbols see text.

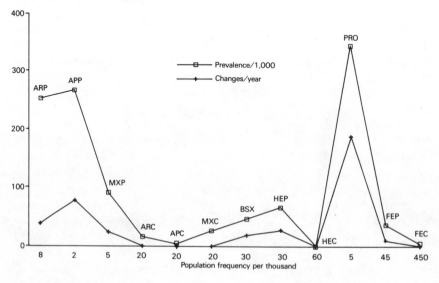

The equilibrium profile

Figure 1 is an example of an AIDS profile and perhaps I can explain what it means. The lower line is the new partner acquisition rate in different behavioural groups, I have called it *a*. The upper line is the prevalence of HIV infection when the system eventually comes to equilibrium. This makes certain assumptions: that nobody changes their behaviour, that people who die are replaced, and a number of others. You will see that there is a correlation between the two lines. The different columns (ie behaviour groups) are labelled and the first three mean:

ARP = anal receptive promiscuous

APP = anal penetrating promiscuous

MXP = mixed promiscuous

As well as these three grades of promiscuous homosexual, we have the same three again but this time *coupled (ARC, APC, MXC)* which means they are **not** promiscuous, although not quite monogamous.

Then we have bisexuals. I have only one sort of bisexual in the profile *(BSX)* but it is possible to think of three different sorts. There is an important question: "What do bisexuals do when they are not at home?". Are they mainly receptive or penetrating? I presumed at first they were probably anal penetrating because that is the direction they think if they are bisexual but maybe they do not go outside to get what they already get at home, so perhaps they behave the other way round. This is the degree of detail which might be very important and on which we do not at present have data.

Finally we have the heterosexual classes, male and female, each divided into promiscuous and non-promiscuous. Female prostitutes are designated separately.

It is possible in this way to divide the population into almost as many classes as you wish. The number is fairly arbitrary but you do have to give each of them a name, you do have to define their contact pattern with other classes, and you do have to declare their frequency within the population. This last point is important because a group with a low prevalence of HIV infection may nevertheless have a high frequency in the population and make an important contribution to the total picture. The contribution is the product of prevalence and frequency. The total picture is then assembled from all these products.

So that is what a profile looks like in general, although it is quite arbitrary in its degree of elaboration of the population, and the number of groups into which it is subdivided. In this profile I have 12 groups but the limit is set only by technical problems such as that of printing it all onto paper.

How did I get to this point? I will explain from the beginning in stages. The computer program incorporates some fairly simple ideas which are really based upon the mass action theory of communicable disease and we trace their development through simple asexual transmission, through the simple heterosexual transmission, to the heterogeneous modes of transmission associated with AIDS.

E G Knox

Asexual transmission

Let us consider the epidemiology of plantar warts, which may be caught asexually, and then extrapolate to sexual transmission in a homogeneous population. If you have plantar warts in swimming baths, you have a population which is divided into two classes, infective and susceptible, and we will call the prevalence of infectives p and of susceptibles $1-p$. There is a net rate of transfer between the two classes with a positive and a negative component, as shown in Figure 2. The negative component represents the people who get better, and it depends upon the decay rate of the infectious stage, D which is the reciprocal of the mean duration of the infective stage. For example if the mean duration of the infective stage is 2 years then D is 0.5 and this is the proportion getting better in a year.

The other component describes transfer in the other direction, from susceptible to infective, and this involves the mass action law. The number of people becoming infective is proportional to the number of susceptibles $1-p$, to the number of infectious people p, to the contact rate a, and to the infectiousness on contact t. (In the case of AIDS, a is the rate of acquisition of new partners and is thus the reciprocal of the mean interval between new partners. We must also then redefine the transfer factor t which is the risk of transferring infection during contact if one partner is infective and the other is susceptible).

Figure 2

The equilibrium prevalence of a communicable disease (see text for key to symbols).

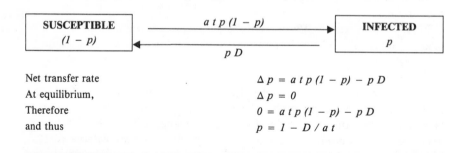

Net transfer rate	$\Delta p = a t p (1 - p) - p D$
At equilibrium,	$\Delta p = 0$
Therefore	$0 = a t p (1 - p) - p D$
and thus	$p = 1 - D / a t$

Returning to the simpler example of plantar warts, if the rate of transfer from susceptible to infected exceeds the rate of transfer in the other direction, we can see that the prevalence will increase until it reaches equilibrium, when the two rates are equal, that is Δp is zero. The zero expression can be simplified as shown, to give an expression for prevalence at equilibrium. We can from this establish that a decay rate D greater than at prevents survival of the disease in the community. On the other hand, values of D between 0 and at allow the disease to survive at a determined equilibrium level.

Heterosexual transmission

If we look now at diseases like syphilis and gonorrhoea, there is the added complexity of two sexes but otherwise the models are similar (Figure 3). The two components of the transfer between the two states are designated as alpha and beta but male values are coded *1* and female values are coded *2*. The two equations look very much the same but note that the boys get infected from the girls and the girls get infected from the boys, so that each equation refers to the prevalence in the other sex. It makes the algebra a bit more complicated but it really is a logical extension of the basic model and we now have expressions for equilibrium prevalences (male and female) for a sexually transmitted disease in a homogeneous population.

Figure 3
The equilibrium prevalence of a chronic disease affecting two sexes.

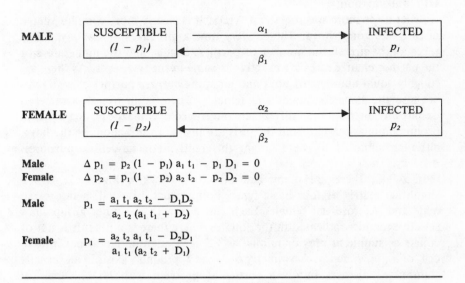

Male $\Delta p_1 = p_2 (1 - p_1) a_1 t_1 - p_1 D_1 = 0$
Female $\Delta p_2 = p_1 (1 - p_2) a_2 t_2 - p_2 D_2 = 0$

Male $p_1 = \dfrac{a_1 t_1 a_2 t_2 - D_1 D_2}{a_2 t_2 (a_1 t_1 + D_2)}$

Female $p_1 = \dfrac{a_2 t_2 a_1 t_1 - D_2 D_1}{a_1 t_1 (a_2 t_2 + D_1)}$

The condition for survival in the heterosexual population is that the partner acquisition rate *a* must conform to the expression in Figure 4. Obviously, if either t_1 or t_2 is zero then the denominator becomes zero and the disease is not sustainable. Note that the values of *t* state the transfer risk for the whole duration of the partnership, not just for one contact. I have inserted some arbitrary figures, which would be reasonably representative (in our present state of knowledge) for the heterosexual transmission of AIDS, and with these figures it would appear that the disease is sustained in that stratum of the population where *a* is greater than 2. Such a stratum clearly exists. The figures shown by Professor Klaus Dietz suggest there is a stratum of the heterosexual population where the value exceeds 6.

There is another stratum of the population in which the infection will not be sustained and this has parallels with the known epidemiology of gonorrhoea. Here there is one stratum where everybody has it (on and off), and another where nobody has it. They mix from time to time and thus the disease spreads. It looks as if this is going to happen for AIDS and such figures as we have or can guess suggest that it will reach an analogous stable equilibrium within a heterogeneous heterosexual population.

Figure 4
The condition for survival of an infection in a heterosexual population (see text).

Condition for survival is	$a > D/(t_1\ t_2)^{0.5}$
For example, given that	$D\ =\ 0.1$ $t_1\ =\ 0.100$ $t_2\ =\ 0.025$
Then survival occurs if	$a > 2$

HIV transmission

Now let us be more specific about AIDS. It is clearly more complex than a disease like gonorrhoea. There, every time a girl takes a new boy, a boy takes a new girl, so the number of partners change and the numerators of the partner change rates are exactly the same in the two sexes. As there are roughly equal numbers of boys and girls, the *average* partner change rates are also the same for males and females. There is an overall symmetry, despite any distributional differences. Averaged overall, the boys are just as promiscuous as the girls and the girls are just as promiscuous as the boys, although some of us were taught differently. For modelling purposes, $a_1\ =\ a_2$.

In AIDS, there are many transmission pathways. Figure 5 gives a simplified matrix of four basic types: homosexual, bisexual, heterosexual male and heterosexual female. Each can mix with the other groups in a selective manner indicated in the squares where there is a plus. It is not of course as simple as **plus** or **minus**, as we need quantitative values in each cell for a_1, a_2, t_1 and t_2. Asymmetry of t_1 and t_2 probably exists in all sexually transmitted diseases but is a particular problem with HIV. Numerical asymmetries in the numbers of persons engaging in the different kinds of partnership also lead to asymmetries between a_1 and a_2. Let us see how this works.

If you have a large army camp that is mainly male, near a small town where just 50% of the population are female, and they mix. Then there is an asymmetry of a. Every time a boy takes a new girl, a girl takes a new boy, so the numerators remain the same but they are shared among **unequal** numbers of poeple so the smaller of the two groups has a higher value of a. This also occurs in prostitution.

There is a particular problem with heterosexual prostitution and its representation within a model. In innocence, or ignorance, I used to think of the anal receptive heterosexual as the prostitute. Now of course there **are** anal receptive prostitutes but I am told that in the more vigorous gay communities, the prostitutes are usually anal penetrative. There are fewer of them, but some of them perform quite heroically at almost unimaginable levels of activity and their values of a are much greater than for their customers. Indeed, until I understood this point, I was at a loss with this model to explain why the majority of the cases has occurred in the anal receptive group. The number of cases is the product of both the prevalence

Figure 5
Simplified matrix of transmission pathways between groups excluding negatives. For symbols see text.

		1	2	3	4
Male homosexual	1	+	+	−	−
Male bisexual	2	+	+	−	+
Male heterosexual	3	−	−	−	+
Female heterosexual	4	−	+	+	−

$$p_j = \sum_{i=1}^{i=4} f_{j.i} \frac{(at)_{j.i}(at)_{i.j} - D_j D_i}{(at)_{i.j}[(at)_{j.i} + D_j]}$$

and the frequency within the population, and a less promiscuous group is by definition the more abundant.

Input to the model
The next issue is that of the data or estimates or even guesses that are to be put into the model. One of the main objectives of creating models is to show what data are really essential for accurate prediction, and to show what data are relatively insensitive, so that a guess will do. The range of values used in the model have been described in the published version[1] and the sources described. They were derived partly from a process of *a priori* ranking within the model, and partly from sporadic pieces of data which were used to calibrate the ranked system.

The values for partner change rates among the different contact-cells of the extended matrix also demanded reconciliation between the assigned behaviour of the "preferers" and the implied preferences of the "preferred". It is necessary to operate a simulated market in preferences in order to reconcile inconsistencies and to render them consistent within a single matrix. In this model I used geometric means to reach a compromise. This was the most difficult element in constructing the model.

Outputs

Table 1 shows an example of some of the results. The equilibrium prevalence comes out overall at about 120 per 1,000 with an equilibrium incidence of about 12 per 1,000 per annum. Another version of the programme introduces a dynamic process, showing how the incidence and prevalence will change from year to year, but this is at present very crude and I have not published it. One can start at a low level and run it year by year, say 20 steps per year, and get an idea of the rate at which the incidence increases. I mention this interim work merely to say that I drew exactly the same general conclusion as the other speakers presenting primarily dynamic models. That is, the more promiscuous groups reach equilibrium fairly quickly, in 10, 15 or 20 years, whereas the incidence in the less promiscuous groups is still increasing after 40, 50 or 60 years. This means that these groups never reach equilibrium because they do not have a sexual lifetime of partner change as long as that. So this is one of the points where the equilibrium model begins to break down, and it does not surprise me that Professor Klaus Dietz, with his more detailed model of heterosexual transmission, gets a higher critical level for disease survival than I do.

Table 1

The incidence and prevalence of HIV at equilibrium by behavioural class. The decay rate of the infectious stage D is set at 0.1 and rates are expressed per 1,000 population.

Behavioural Class	Incidence	Prevalence
1. M. Hom. AR-Promiscuous	83.39	833.86
2. M. Hom. AP-Promiscuous	83.44	834.37
3. M. Hom. AP/AR-Promiscuous	64.13	641.28
4. M. Hom. AR-Coupled	25.29	252.95
5. M. Hom. AP-Coupled	3.93	39.33
6. M. Hom. AP/AR Coupled	34.78	347.79
7. M. Bisexual	41.42	414.16
8. M. Het. Promiscuous	51.12	511.18
9. M. Het. Not Promiscuous	1.51	15.13
10. F. Prostitute	91.05	910.46
11. F. Promiscuous	57.59	575.88
12. F. Not Promiscuous	6.64	66.45
Total	**12.05**	**120.48**

The kind of answer we are getting for HIV in this country would mean 20,000 to 40,000 deaths from AIDS per year at equilibrium, assuming that 15 per cent of the people with HIV infection will come down with AIDS. This proportion may well prove to be much higher.

Dynamic and age-dependent modelling

I will finish by indicating the directions in which modelling techniques are likely to move. In addition to the development of dynamic models operating across the full matrix of behaviour types, I believe that the other important element to be incorporated is the matrix of contact between different age-groups within each of these behaviour-type compartments.

I did a study some years ago on papilloma virus transmission in relation to cervical cancer. In this model, because I only had male and female groups, I was able to elaborate in another direction. The model was broken down by age. At equilibrium there is an accumulating prevalence of infection with age so it matters very much who mixes with whom in these terms. Thus, a new cohort of 15 year olds or 16 year olds starting out on their sexual careers can be as promiscuous as they like as long as they stick to their own cohort. The cohort will remain uninfected and the disease will eventually wash out at the top end of the population. If they are totally *indiscriminate* and mix with older people, then the younger cohorts will be infected by the older cohorts. In real life the degree of mixing between age-groups is determined again by market preferences.

Data on parenthood show a correlation of about 0.6 between ages, and values around this level were used in the exploration of papilloma virus transmission. The preference correlation interacted with a. The less age discrimination the population shows, the smaller are the values of a needed to exceed the threshold at which the disease will survive. It is therefore important to incorporate this aspect of behaviour within future HIV models. Indeed, it is not even as simple as that. There is also the issue of sexual career evolution and the manner in which different behaviour types change with age. This is not just a question of changing frequencies of partner change, but a question of qualitative changes in patterns of sexual practice. The modelling problems yet to be solved, and the data yet to be collected, are going to be exceedingly important for understanding a disease in which the main stream of transmission at equilibrium is likely to be in younger age groups exhibiting very fluid patterns of sexual relationship.

Reference

1. *Knox EG*
   A transmission model for AIDS
   European J Epidem 1986; **2**; 165–177

Paper 6

Professor Sir David Cox
Imperial College, University of London

Estimation of the incubation period and data needs

Chairman, Ladies and Gentlemen: I am odd man out here, in that the centre of my research interest is quite far from the topics being discussed today. I am going first to do what I have been asked to, namely to talk briefly about the analysis of some data on incubation period. Then, if there is time, I will come briefly to the question of the sort of data it would be good to have.

The incubation period

So far as I know, rather few sets of data with clearly defined instants of infection and of development of AIDS are available. The data I am going to describe were very kindly supplied to Professor Roy Anderson by Dr Peterman of the Centers for Disease Control, Atlanta. This is a chance to thank him for the data and to apologise for not having discussed the analysis with him. The excuse is that the analysis was only completed a day or so ago! There are data on 299 transfusion-associated AIDS cases. There is an analysis of some of the individuals reported by Lui and co-authors[1] last year but I think that was on a substantially smaller set of data. A fuller account of the present analysis has been prepared.[2]

The structure of the data is as follows. Individuals are identified as having AIDS, so we are starting retrospectively. The date of transfusion is identified relatively well, and taken as the time origin for all calculations. The sex and the age at transfusion are the explanatory variables or risk factors.

The date of transfusion goes from 1978 to 1984, with the majority of cases towards the end of this period. Think of the 1984 transfusion cases; for these individuals the elapsed time to the development of AIDS must be quite short because the construction of the data is closed in 1986 and there is no possibility of any longer time showing. On the other hand, for those who were transfused in 1978 there is potentially a much longer period of exposure to risk following transfusion. If one just took incubation times to development of AIDS as they stand, that would be quite misleading. Also there are no data on those exposed to risk who did not develop AIDS.

Thus a fairly sophisticated analysis is needed. We used a rather different method from that used by Lui and I am not going to explain technical detail. I should stress before continuing that there is no information in these data about the proportion of those transfused who ever develop AIDS. There is no information whether the curve is levelling off at 30%, 50%,

70% or 100% simply because people who were infected at transfusion but never developed the disease will never appear in these data.

The analysis is joint work with Professor Roy Anderson, Professor Billard and Mr Graham Medley[2] who has done the computational work, which is decidedly non-trivial. First we postulated that the number exposed to risk was growing either linearly or exponentially over the time period in question. We fitted various models and the first conclusion was that the exponential model seemed to fit substantially better than the linear model, and that the doubling time of this exponential growth was about a year. This is a conclusion coming at the end of an intricate calculation; it is not a direct consequence of the data, and the fact that the time of one year fits in rather well with other kinds of data is a suggestion that the analysis is meaningful. The main conclusion is that the fitted distribution of incubation times has a median of about 5 years and a very long tail extending to 10 years and beyond.

The data were split into roughly equal numbers of men and women. We fitted the curves separately to men and women; there was no major difference. Then there was a split based on age; 36 patients under 5 years gave a curve coming to a maximum at about 2 years, whereas the curve for all the remainder came to a maximum at about 6 years. This is strong evidence, therefore, not that the very young patients are necessarily more at risk, but rather that those who do develop AIDS do so much more quickly than older patients.

Data needed

In considering general points about the kind of data that it would be good to see collected, I must make the disclaimer that it would be pretentious for a statistician to say precisely what data must be collected. Obviously many considerations enter. On the other hand statistical methods are involved, not only in the analysis of data, but equally importantly in the collection of data, and there are principles of study design whose consideration is crucial if effort is to be spent economically. Therefore, I offer some tentative comments and have classified them into those concerned with:

  a. monitoring or surveillance;

  b. collecting biological parameters; and

  c. sociological aspects of sexual behaviour;

although it is perhaps rather artifical to regard **c** as different from the biological parameters.

For **surveillance** one wants to see the number of AIDS cases, measures of seropositivity (both in higher risk groups and in the population as a whole), and the reaction to publicity campaigns. It has been suggested that any large Government programme should spend 5% of its money on monitoring what goes on. I do not know where the figure of 5% came from, but some non-trivial amount of effort should surely be spent, in particular on monitoring the impact of advertising campaigns. Professor Anderson has already commented on this. We must try to look deeply into the possible effects of these campaigns; asking superficial questions is unlikely to be adequate.

For the **biological parameters,** the enormous dispersion of the distribution of the incubation period raises the question of what are the explanatory variables that control whether the period is small or large. Connected partly with that are the determinants of the seriousness of the illness itself, while full AIDS develops or various associated conditions, and what determines the passage into one of these states rather than another. Investigations connected with determinants of infectivity are clearly of great importance and difficulty.

Coming to rather more technical points, the case-control study is a widely used technique in epidemiology and is likely to be appropriate for AIDS particularly in studies of those infected who may or may not progress to AIDS. There are techniques that have been developed for answering sensitive questions whilst preserving anonymity for the subjects such as the so-called randomised response method developed in connection with surveys of abortion at a time when **knowledge** of the occurrence of an abortion was a potentially criminal offence. This is an ingenious idea for getting people to answer sensitive questions whilst preserving their anonymity from the investigator as well as from anyone else. Its practicality is unclear.

There is a final more general question concerning empirical prediction versus model-based prediction. There is surely a role for both. In the very short term, empirical prediction methods are valuable but should we not be looking for the middle ground: the empirical prediction that brings in certain information from model-based considerations, and empirical prediction for particular countries that also uses data from other countries. This is necessary because the amount of data is so small that confidence bands for the prediction could be substantially narrowed by intelligent use of all the data that is available. I was very impressed by the CDC work that we heard this morning. They have the largest quantity of data but in making predictions for our particular country, we need to use USA and other experience whilst not assuming that everything is going to be exactly the same as it is in the USA. This raises interesting technical statistical issues.

References

1. *Lui KJ, Lawrence DN and Morgan WM*
   A model-based approach for mean incubation period of transfusion-associated acquired immunodeficiency syndrome
   Proc Nat Acad Sci 1986; **83**; 3051–3055

2. *Medley GF, Anderson RM, Cox DR and Billard L*
   The incubation period of Acquired Immune Deficiency Syndrome (AIDS) in patients infected via blood transfusion
   Nature 1987; **328**; 718–721

Questions

Dr Mann

I would like to ask whether there is any evidence that the distribution of incubation periods might differ for persons infected through transfusion from that for persons infected sexually?

Sir David Cox

I do not know of quantitative data that bear on this.

Dr Mann

There is the data emerging from the Control Board studies suggesting increasing risk and even rising risks with time.

Dr Meade Morgan

I will comment on that very briefly. We have compared the data from Dr Lui's work with a similar analysis of the San Fancisco Control Board data but the numbers were not large enough to show a statistical difference between the two distribution times. However the more recent data from the Board suggest an increasing hazard with time.

Professor Anderson

Implicit in the Weibull distribution that David Cox used is the assumption that a hazard function increases either linearly or faster with time. If one looks in more detail at other parts of that transfusion data, then in fact one can show that the probability of converting to AIDS rises more steeply through time than linearly.

Question

In your list of data needed, the column of social behaviour was left empty and previous speakers, Professor Anderson in particular, have stressed the need for studies of sexual behaviour. I am wondering whether you are inclined to agree with them that there is a real need for data on sexual behaviour? For example, the frequency of bisexual behaviour and what they get up to.

Sir David Cox

This seems quite crucial and the data should be of high quality and in as much detail as is feasible. Also its statistical specification would have to be quite complicated bringing in age dependence, transition between different schemes of behaviour and so forth. I simply left the column blank through a feeling that this was an artificial distinction from other biological parameters.

Question

If I may just continue, Professor Anderson made the point that there is an urgent need for this information and this might well be the case especially as the education programmes must depend on it. We need to have a base line on the sexual activity of the population now, and then see how it changes.

Sir David Cox

I agree. Could I add one point on a different issue that I did not mention when I was speaking. When the data were sent to us, we were concerned with the possibility of changing patterns of diagnosis. Mathematically, it is possible to build this factor into the model, but so far at least, the data do not seem extensive enough for this to be useful.

Dr Meade Morgan

Have you calculated any confidence limits on the mean incubation times. Again one of the problems in the Lui paper was that he estimated the mean at 5 years with a 90% range between 3 and 13 years.

Sir David Cox

It is simply because there are no data whatever in the tail of the distribution so that the mean is very ill-defined and is probably not the right summary parameter.

Question

One of the aspects people consider in relation to incubation period and chance of getting the disease is that other infections are acquired at the same time, which may be cofactors particularly in the homosexuals. You probably do not have enough cases, but is there any evidence of an effect from the reason why the subjects had blood transfusion upon the probability that they actually develop infection? There are of course two likely groups, the elderly who are ill for some reason, and younger subjects who may have received blood transfusion for trauma.

Sir David Cox

It is important to try and put into the model as many potential explanatory factors as possible to try to cut down the enormous so-far unexplained dispersion.

Dr Peterman

There are some studies that are looking for cofactors in the adult transfusion recipients, but these are limited studies on a limited number of people and they have not found anything so far. I think the difference in the incubation period for the children is due to the fact that almost all of these children are newborn and they have quite different immune systems from the adults.

David Cox

Paper 7

Dr Jonathan Mann
World Health Organisation, Geneva

The World Health Organisation approach to the global problem of AIDS
There are two parallels that can be drawn between the smallpox epidemic
and the current AIDS pandemic. Firstly, the World Health Organization
(WHO) has made a commitment to the prevention and control of AIDS that
equals and will surpass the commitment it made to the eradication of
smallpox. Secondly, the eradication of smallpox was accomplished by the
application of a strategy based on epidemiological assessment rather than
by vaccination of the entire world population.

AIDS, however, is a far more complex problem than was smallpox. In
this regard, I will outline a perspective from WHO about our ability to
predict, forecast and assess the shape of this epidemic. We must remember
that we are still, in historical terms, only at the beginning of the worldwide
epidemic of human immunodeficiency virus (HIV) infection and AIDS.

These are phases in the evolution of our perception of AIDS. The first
phase was awareness. It was characterised by what we might call *parachute
epidemiology*, — researchers could parachute into developing countries,
collect some samples, and leave. This results in some data but not much
understanding. Parachute epidemiology was important, however, because it
increased our awareness of the global scope of the HIV and AIDS problem.
As a result, 99 countries have now officially reported cases of AIDS to
WHO (by August 1987 this figure had increased to 122 countries).

The second phase of our collective encounter with AIDS started with the
first actions, — actions to control an epidemic which was not yet well
understood. Apart from protecting the blood supply, these first actions
focussed on changing sexual behaviour. Early on, male homosexual
communities in various countries were nearly alone in initiating educational campaigns aimed at changing sexual behaviour. Now, increasingly,
countries are following the lead of the United Kingdom campaign "Don't
die of ignorance" and large-scale educational campaigns directed to the
general public are underway throughout the world.

Data from Brazil suggest that such programmes can stimulate behavioural change as well as increased awareness and knowledge about AIDS. In
February 1987 a large survey was conducted in São Paolo where most of the
cases of AIDS in Brazil have occurred. Of a sample of approximately 500
males aged 15−25 years, 52% claimed that they frequently visited female
prostitutes. In the past 16 months however, about two-thirds of these men
have stopped having contact with prostitutes, and about 30% have reduced

the frequency of their visits. The prostitutes themselves have verified these responses, as over two-thirds reported a decline, often substantial, in the number of customers.

The third phase in our perception of AIDS has come with the realisation that we are lacking valuable data about sexual practices. To obtain these data, we must first educate the researchers. During the last few years, those involved in AIDS research have learned a great deal about bisexual behaviour, homosexual behaviour, and intravenous drug use.

We need to know the distribution in the population of various sexual practices and the role that certain practices may play in amplifying epidemics. We need to do more research on the transmission dynamics of the human immunodeficiency virus and on risk factors for its transmission. We need to know more about the incidence of disease in different populations. Data from Zaire suggest that the acquisition of HIV antibody during a one-year period was a little less than 1% in a reasonably large open population of heterosexuals.

We need to know more about virology and its practical application to the biology of HIV transmission. Are the viruses different in different places? Are there differences in molecular structure that translate into differences in terms of transmission or transmissibility? Exactly how is the virus transmitted? When is the virus transmitted and why is it sometimes not transmitted? For example, in some studies of spouses of HIV-infected persons with haemophilia, there are very low rates of transmission, despite what appears to be more than adequate opportunity for infection.

Now, in 1987, we are beginning to enter a fourth phase in which a conceptual model of the epidemiology and transmission of AIDS is being developed. This model will allow us to develop interventions which we can subsequently assess. The role of intervention studies is critical because whatever the epidemiology, only population-based intervention studies can prove whether our proposed cause-and-effect relationships are valid.

We need also to consider intervention studies in the context of the availability of additional tools, such as therapeutic agents or vaccines. If drugs that reduce infectiousness become available, there will be other ways of intervening to prevent HIV transmission.

Other problems exist. We now have HIV-2 in addition to HIV-1. Moreover, HIV-3, HIV-4, and a series of other retroviruses are yet to be discovered. At WHO we are beginning to reconceptualise our ideas about AIDS. The *Special Programme on AIDS* will eventually become in essence a *Retroviral Programme*. Evidence is emerging that there are interactions among the retroviruses which will complicate our model and our predictions.

There are also interactions with other diseases. For example, genital ulcer disease, particularly chancroid, may be associated with an increased risk of transmission of HIV. In other words, the concomitant chancroid may be a risk factor for transmission, so that the distribution of chancroid in a population may be a critical variable in the development of a model focussing on transmission.

In addition to disease interactions, data on heterosexual populations in

Africa and male homosexual populations in the West suggest that there are factors that may interfere with the integrity of the epithelial barrier to HIV. Thus, in studies of male homosexuals, rectal douching before intercourse, and, in prostitutes in Zaire, the insertion of a variety of products into the vagina on a regular basis, were practices associated with increased risks of infection.

What is the World Health Organization doing in terms of modelling and conceptualizing the problem? We are extremely concerned about the present dearth of reliable tools to estimate the current size of this epidemic, or to predict its future course. Therefore, we are all in jeopardy of overstating or understating the relevant issues. The *Special Programme on AIDS* will convene a consultation of the many groups that are working on modelling. The consultation will seek to establish communication and exchange of ideas among epidemiologists, virologists, clinicians, public health officials, modellers and statisticians, and thus avoid the dangers of each group working in isolation.

In closing, the critical role of international collaboration should be emphasised. We must assume that there will be no vaccine or treatment within the next few years. This assumption places us squarely before our dilemma. With no vaccine or treatment, a conceptual understanding is vital to guide our public health efforts. AIDS is a pandemic, yet there are places in the world at different phases in its evolution; international collaboration must bring out the best that science, medicine and public health have to offer.

Questions

Question

In the global view you are able to take, are there differences in the epidemics in different countries which are such as to make you believe that the experience of one country is unlikely to be useful as a guide to the epidemic in other countries? Perhaps you are able to group countries so that you might imagine that the epidemic in one may resemble that in others in the group.

Dr Mann

I do not think we can answer because even among European countries there are such dramatic differences among AIDS cases, differences in the distribution of risk factors, in reporting, and to some extent in analysis. Outside the European region, we know of some countries where there are a very small number of reported intravenous drug-using AIDS patients. However, in some of these countries, a physician who treats an intravenous drug abuser is legally required to report him immediately to the police. This legal requirement must influence reporting and exchange of information. So, unfortunately, it is the lack of comparable data that prevents us from making much more than anecdotal observations.

Dr Reid

Just as a follow-up to that question, could I ask if you have any feel for evidence of transmission across national boundaries, because what is in one country might spread to another? I am thinking here of the fact that about 9 million people go abroad each year from this country, many of them for package holidays and package holidaymakers sometimes may be promiscuous. Is there evidence from WHO data of infection being taken back because package tours are now going to Gambia and also to Kenya?

Dr Mann
I am glad that you focussed on the nationals who leave their countries and return. People usually look only at the danger that those outside may appear to create to those inside. There are many reports of expatriates, usually European men, who visit other countries and become infected through readily-identifiable modes of transmission. Their small number, when contrasted with the endemic epidemiology of the disease in countries such as the United Kingdom and France, leads to the impression that this travel does not contribute substantially to a national epidemic.

It may be different in some parts of Asia where the number of infected persons appears to be much lower. This brings us to the subject of international travel and HIV infection, which a WHO consultation addressed in Geneva from 2–3 March 1987. Because of the extraordinary logistic and operational problems associated with any effort to screen travellers, such as the "window period" in serological testing, the consultation concluded that any effort to reduce the risk in one's own country through screening of travellers would be at extraordinary cost and, if it succeeded at all, would slow only slightly the dissemination of the virus.

Professor Healy
I wanted to ask about the African situation where it appears that the sex ratio is roughly one to one and newspaper reports suggest that the same is true of the black population in New York. Does anybody know if this is virological or sociological or both?

Dr Mann
I have not heard that statistic for New York, but I will defer to my colleagues from Atlanta. The assumption that most people are making so far is that differences observed between groups within a country are related more closely to behavioural factors rather than to intrinsic differences in susceptibility. However, this has not been completely worked out, nor has the issue of the virus identity in different parts of the world.

Dr Meade Morgan
I do not have the figures with me on the male-to-female ratio among infected blacks in New York City, but we know that the major risk factor among blacks in that area is intravenous drug abuse so that could easily explain the equal ratio.

Professor Anderson
In European countries and America, we have estimates of the doubling time of AIDS cases and we know of some excellent studies of seroprevalence in

African countries. Is there any longitudinal data yet to hint at the doubling time in the heterosexual population from any African country?

Dr Mann
The only data we have, from which we have not calculated a doubling time, but which are essentially the same information expressed a different way, involve the sero-acquisition studies in two populations in Zaire. The published data show a sero-acquisition rate of 0.75% per annum. Sero-acquisition at 1% per annum, based on a background seroprevalence of about 6% in those populations, gives an estimate of doubling time which would certainly be longer than that in the other populations mentioned.

Sir Donald Acheson
I wanted to ask Professor Knox if he would reconsider the use of the words "promiscuous" and "promiscuity" in the interests of science. It seems to me that there is a difficulty in that they mean something different to everybody and we ought to replace them with quantitative estimates.

Professor Knox
Yes. The variable a is the quantity of acquisition that I used because I was trying to pretend that the population was not homosexually mixing and that it classified itself into different qualitative behaviour groups. Within each of these are different general levels, and it is therefore an attempt to divide the population qualitatively and then quantitatively within each qualitative group. That is why I used the word.

Dr Tyrrell
I had a question which I think is very important and arises from what Dr Mann said. I have been asked questions in India about what was happening and what should be done. I am very concerned with this approach, which I know is good science, that we should wait and get the data thoroughly established and do our calculations properly. When I see the fuse burning rapidly in a country like India which is quickly getting to the point where the sort of measures it could reasonably take will be unable to cope with the scale of the problem.

I wonder whether Dr Mann would like to temper this point "let us do it thoroughly and take a long time over it" with some discretion as in certain circumstances interim and partial answers will have to be used. It is rather like my father in business having to say: "I know that if I wait until next Friday *The Economist* will tell me why everything happened the way it did, but meantime I have to get the factory going and sell something!" It is a matter of human affairs, not simple scientific certainty.

Dr Mann
Thank you very much for giving me the chance to clarify this point if it did not come through in my talk because I was so concerned about the long term. We are also very interested in what happens in the short term. The initial efforts that concern us are to educate people, to induce behaviour

change, and, in the case of places like Africa and South America, to implement the blood tranfusion screening that already is taken for granted in other parts of the world. That is all absolutely critical and has to be done.

Chairman

I think the message from this morning is that the mathematical models are not yet able to take us very far into the future. Perhaps short-term prediction is all that is possible now, and there is a great deal of work to be done on the epidemiology, on the biology and on the social factors influencing AIDS. I do not think that we can go much further until lunch!

———————————— End of Second Session ————————————

Third Session

Chairman Dr David Tyrrell
Chairman of the Working Party on AIDS
Medical Research Council

Paper 8

Dr Spence Galbraith
Director, Communicable Diseases Surveillance Centre
Public Health Laboratory Service, England & Wales

The shape of the United Kingdom epidemic

Introduction

The purpose of this paper is to present the methods of AIDS surveillance in the United Kingdom and the findings to the end of February 1987.

It is hard to believe that it was only just over 5 years ago that the description of the first case in the United Kingdom was published in the *Lancet*[1] in December 1981. Following this publication CDSC set up a surveillance programme based on three methods of data collection, using the case definition of the Centers for Disease Control, Atlanta. First, copies of death entries referring to AIDS and Kaposi's sarcoma were provided to CDSC by the Office of Population Censuses and Surveys. Second, laboratory reports from medical microbiologists sent to CDSC, initially of opportunistic infections for which there was no apparent cause but later, after the discovery of the causative virus and the development of HIV antibody tests, also of positive tests. Third, and perhaps the most important, an arrangement from 1982 for reporting by clinicians to CDSC, initially mainly by genito-urinary physicians. In addition to these three methods of data collection, a special study was set up to monitor the serological status and health of health-care staff accidentally exposed to HIV infection during their work.

Methods

The laboratory reporting system

A routine national laboratory reporting system has been in existence in England and Wales since 1939 and this includes the reporting of opportunistic infections. Thus in 1982 all that was necessary was to ask laboratories to indicate on the reports whether or not there was any apparent cause for immunosuppression. If the opportunistic infection was thought to be associated with AIDS then laboratories were asked to indicate details including risk group. When HIV antibody tests became available these were included in the same reporting system and a special form of report was added to the system containing data on age, sex, risk group and clinical condition.

The clinical reporting system

The clinical reporting system was a new development and was established initially by writing to all dermatologists and genito-urinary physicians personally, inviting them to report in strictest confidence to the medical director of CDSC, cases of AIDS and suspected AIDS. Subsequently genito-urinary physicians have been sent a personal letter each year reminding them of the need to report cases of AIDS and information was provided for all doctors by publications in the *British Medical Journal* and *Lancet*, and by letters from the Chief Medical Officer. More recently close links with community physicians in district and regional health authorities have been developed in order to promote and validate the reporting system. The system involves the completion of a questionnaire by the clinician concerned who then sends it to CDSC or the Scottish Unit by confidential mail. On arrival the envelopes are opened, the forms given serial numbers and dates, and then filed in a secure cabinet by the current month. Each week the forms are inspected by a group consisting of a clinician, an epidemiologist and a statistician and the forms are coded and checked before **unnamed** data are entered into a microcomputer. The data are then verified and checked for duplicates. Standard monthly tabulations are produced and other tabulations in response to ad hoc enquiries.

Results

Cases of AIDS

Until the end of February 1987 altogether 731 cases had been reported to CDSC or to the Scottish Unit, 377 of which had died. These reports in 3-monthly periods from 1982 are shown in Figure 1. There has been an

Figure 1
Cumulative quarterly total of new cases of AIDS reported to the CDSC and the CD(S)U

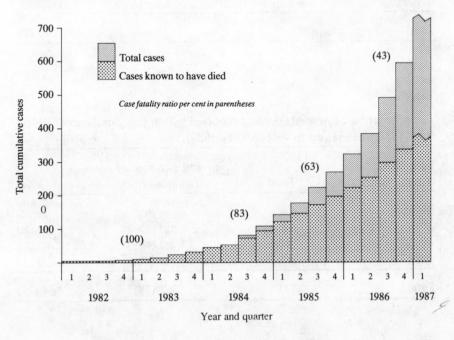

exponential increase with a doubling in number of cases about every 10 months. The case-fatality rate until the end of 1983 was 100%. In 1984 it was 83%, in 1985 it was 63%, and in 1986 it was 43%; the overall case-fatality rate being about 50%.

The epidemic has been largely confined to the London area; Table 1 shows the distribution by regional health authority and it can be seen that the four Thames regions make up nearly 80% of all cases. Unlike the information reported from the United States, the proportion reported from the four Thames regions has not changed significantly with time (Table 2). Most of the homosexual cases (82%) were reported from the four Thames regions (Table 3) whereas only 45% of the cases in other risk-groups were reported from these regions.

Table 1

The distribution of AIDS cases by Regional Health Authority (reports up to 28 February 1987).

Region	Cases	Deaths	Region	Cases	Deaths
Northern	20	14	Oxford	6	4
Yorkshire	9	4	S. Western	10	8
Trent	12	7	W. Midlands	15	12
E. Anglia	5	3	Mersey	10	10
NW Thames	363	165	N. Western	31	16
NE Thames	130	60	Wales	11	9
SE Thames	59	30	Scotland	16	11
SW Thames	15	10	N. Ireland	3	3
Wessex	16	11			
Total				**731**	**377**

Table 2

The proportion of new AIDS cases reported within the four Thames RHAs from 1982 to 1987 (up to 28 February 1987).

Year of report	Total	No. and per cent of cases Thames regions	Other
1982–84	106	85 (80)	21 (20)
1985	164	127 (77)	37 (23)
1986	329	252 (77)	77 (23)
1987	132	103 (78)	29 (22)
Total	**731**	**567 (78)**	**164 (22)**

Table 3

The geographical distribution of AIDS cases arising in homosexuals or bisexuals.

National Health Service region of reporting	Number and per cent of cases	
	Homo-or bisexual	Other
Thames	526 (82)	41 (45)
Wessex/S. Western	17 (3)	9 (10)
Other regions:		
The Midland & North	82 (13)	26 (29)
Wales	2 (1)	9 (10)
Scotland	11 (2)	5 (5)
N. Ireland	2 (1)	1 (1)
Total	**640 (100)**	**91 (100)**

The transmission characteristics of the patients are shown in Table 4, nearly 90% of reported cases have been in homosexual or bisexual men, and so far there have been only 25 cases where the infection was thought to have been acquired heterosexually. The distribution of these patient transmission characteristics have not altered with time (Table 5). However, what has changed is contact between the homosexual cases and North America, many of the cases admitting sexual contact with Americans whilst visiting the United States. In 1982 around 70% of the cases had such overseas contacts whilst in 1986 this proportion had fallen to less than half.

Table 4

New AIDS cases by transmission characteristic.

Transmission characteristic	Number of Cases			
	Male	Female	Total	Deaths
Homosexual/bisexual	640	—	640	317
IV drug abuser	8	2	10	4
Homosexual + IVDA	8	—	8	4
Haemophiliac	28	—	28	22
Recipient of Blood	7	5	12*	10
Heterosexual Contact	14	11	25+	15
Child of HIV+ mother	3	4	7	4
Other	—	1	1	1
Total	**708**	**23**	**731**	**377**

* 8 abroad   +20 abroad

Table 5

New AIDS cases by transmission characteristic from 1982 to 1987 (up to 28 February 1987).

Year of report	Total	No. and per cent of cases	
		Homosexual	Other
1982–84	106	92 (87)	14 (13)
1985	164	145 (88)	19 (12)
1986	329	288 (88)	41 (12)
1987	132	115 (87)	17 (13)
Total	**731**	**640 (88)**	**91 (12)**

Table 6

The transmission characteristic of new AIDS cases thought to have been acquired heterosexually.

Place of infection	Number of cases		
	Male	Female	Total
Probably UK	1	4	5
Probably abroad			
Sexually active Africa	5	4	9
Sexually active elsewhere	2	2	4
Sexual activity unknown	1*	1*	2
Visited UK for treatment	5+	0	5
Total	**14**	**11**	**25**

* Africa   + 4 Africa, 1 Mid. East

Turning to the 25 cases which were thought to have acquired the infection heterosexually (Table 4), only in 5 of these did it seem likely that they acquired the infection in the UK, one male and four females (Table 6). The remaining 20 were thought to have acquired the infection in other countries including 5 who came to this country for diagnosis and treatment. The 5 cases infected in the UK were: the wife of a seropositive haemophiliac, a female prostitute with multiple US contacts, a male who had multiple sexual partners including prostitutes and had shared shaving razors with drug abusers, a female who had sexual contact with several black Africans and a female who had sexual contact with a seropositive intravenous drug abuser.

The fourth case, the female contact of several black Africans, was the only case who did not have contact with a known risk-group. That is of course if black Africans themselves are not regarded as a risk-group, and it is only this one case which could conceivably indicate spread heterosexually outside the accepted risk-groups in this country.

HIV antibody reports
The laboratory reports of positive HIV antibody tests began at the end of 1984 and at first only about half the reports contained any information

Table 7

Reports of positive laboratory tests for HIV antibody for England, Wales & N Ireland.

Time period	Total	Antibody positive reports No. and per cent: risk group not stated
to 31 Dec 1985	1,683	400 (24)
1 Jan to 31 Dec 1986	2,193	185 (8)
1 Jan to 28 Feb 1987	306	38 (12)
Total	**4,182***	**623 (15)**

* 3,957 M, 195 F, 30 NK.

Table 8

Positive laboratory reports of HIV antibody where transmission was thought to have occurred heterosexually, classified by the risk-group involved.

Likely source of infection	Number of persons infected		
	Male	Female	Total
'Risk' groups			
Bisexual	—	5	5 ⎫
IV drug abuser	2	7	9 ⎪
Haemophiliac	—	17	17 ⎬ 36
Transfusion Recipient	—	1	1 ⎪
Prostitute	4	—	4 ⎭
No 'risk' group			
Infected UK	4	2	6 ⎫ 93
Infected abroad	53	34	87 ⎭
Not known	1	5	6
Total	**64**	**71**	**135**

about risk-group. In the period until the end of February 1985, 24% of the reports had no information about risk-groups but this has now fallen substantially. In 1986 only 8% had no information about risk-groups and this is likely to fall further in 1987 as reports with missing data are followed up (Table 7).

Until the end of February 1987 there were 135 HIV antibody positive reports out of total of over 4,000 in which there was evidence that the infection had been heterosexually acquired. Of these, 36 had had sexual contact with individuals in known risk-groups listed in Table 8. The other 99 comprised 6 in which the source of infection was unknown and 87 in which it was likely that the infection was acquired overseas (of which 84 had visited sub-Saharan Africa). Thus, in only 6 did it seem likely that the infection was acquired in the UK. Two of these 6 were female prostitutes and could themselves be regarded as a risk-group, 3 were males who had multiple sexual partners (but there was nothing known about the possible risk group of these partners), and the sixth was a male who had a seropositive consort who was not in a risk-group and this again could possibly indicate spread outside the sexual contacts of recognised risk-groups in this country.

Accidental transmission
There were four reports in the world literature of accidental transmission within households which are listed in Table 9. The first of these was a female in the UK who was a housewife and where it was thought that she was infected by transfer of the virus from a AIDS patient whom she nursed at home, through her weeping eczematous skin lesions. The second was a child who had received vitamin injections with the same needle as a seropositive sibling. The third was the mother of a seriously ill child who was seropositive and it seemed likely that the mother became infected by contamination with blood. The fourth was a brother of a seropositive child where spread was thought possible to have occurred by a bite.

Table 9

Cases of HIV infection where accidental household transmission was thought to be involved.

Person infected	Exposure
F Housewife; U.K. 1985	Home care for AIDS patient. Had skin lesions. CDR 85/42.
M Sibling; Dominica 1985	Shared needle with HIV positive sibling for vitamin injections. Lancet 1986; ii: 627.
F Mother; USA 1986	Home care for seropositive child. MMWR 1986; 35: 76–9.
M Sibling; FDR. 1986	Household contact with seropositive brother. Lancet 1986; ii: 694.

Table 10

Accidental exposure of UK health-care staff to HIV infection: surveillance up to 28 February 1987. There were no seroconversions in this group.

Type of injury	Number of injuries				
	Nurse	Doctor	Lab. wkr.	Other	Total
Needle-stick	28	14	2	9	53
Other sharp	11	7	0	5	23
Splashes	18	6	0	0	24
Aerosols	0	0	2	3	5
Other	34	5	4	2	45
Total	**91**	**32**	**8**	**19**	**150**

Table 11

Confirmed cases of seroconversion in health-care staff world-wide by type of incident.

Person infected	Exposure
F Nurse U.K. 1984	Needle-stick + injection. Lancet 1984; ii: 1376–7.
F Nurse USA 1984	Deep IM needle-stick. NEJM 1986; 314: 1115.
F Nurse Martinique 1985	Superficial needle-stick. Lancet 1986; ii: 814.
F Nurse France 1986	Needle-stick with infected pleural fluid. NEJM 1986; 315: 582

It seems likely, however, that there is a greater risk of accidental transmission in the health care staff caring for infected patients. In the UK the health care staff surveillance scheme has so far included 150 exposed staff with a median follow-up period of 9 months with no seroconversions (Table 10). As will be seen, needlestick injuries in doctors and nurses acounted for a high proportion of the total, many of which were probably preventable. There was one needlestick injury which led to seroconversion in the UK before the survey began; in this case, a nurse, the injury resulted in the injection of blood. So far the four incidents listed in Table 11 are the only confirmed seroconversions in health care staff world-wide. It seems that the risk of infection to these staff is very low and that amongst household contacts who are not sexual contacts even lower still.

Conclusion

The UK surveillance scheme, with all its deficiencies, has at least defined the main transmission routes of HIV infection in this country and has provided sound data on which preventive programmes have been based and will provide data on which they can be evaluated.

Reference

1. *du Bois RM, Branthwaite MA, Mikhail JR and Batten JC*
   Primary *Pneumocystis carinii* and cytomegalovirus infections
   Lancet 1981; **ii**; 1339.

Dr Brian McClelland
Director South East Regional Centre
Scottish National Blood Transfusion Service

HIV Infection in drug-abusers in Scotland
Dr Tyrrell, Ladies and Gentlemen, for several years workers in the United States and in some European countries have been aware that drug misuse was contributing to the spread of HIV infection. This has been reflected in the substantial proportion of AIDS cases in which drug abuse appears to have played a part (Table 1). In Europe, the proportion of drug-related AIDS cases varies widely. The latest WHO figures show that in Italy and Spain approximately 50% of all cases of AIDS appear to be associated with drug use and over the whole of Europe the proportion has risen from 7% at the end of 1985 to 14% at the end of 1986.

Table 1

Data for Scotland from August 1983 to December 1986 showing HIV antibody positives by behavioural class.

	Male	Female	Total	%
Homosexual Bisexual M	152	—	152	15
Drug Misuser	402	211	618	61
Other	149	61	238	24

Total 1,008

This problem came into prominence in the United Kingdom in November 1985 with the publication of a letter in the *Lancet* by John Peutherer[2] and his colleagues in Edinburgh, reporting that 38% of a small series of stored serum samples from drug misusers in Edinburgh contained the HIV antibody. This observation (and in everything else I want to talk about this afternoon) is the work of colleagues in Scotland and I would particularly like to acknowledge their assistance in preparing this talk. I want to try and pick out some salient features of the data which are rapidly accumulating about the epidemic of HIV in Scottish drug misusers concentrating on three aspects which I hope will help in making predictions about the course of the epidemic:

1. How big is the problem of injecting drug use?

2. How prevalent is HIV infection among injecting drug users and how is this epidemic evolving in Scotland?

3. What have we learned so far about the spread from drug abusers to non-drug users?

The first task, and the first rock on which the epidemiologist may founder, is to define the population of drug misusers who are at risk from the use of potentially contaminated needles, syringes, mixing equipment etc. This critical question is very difficult to approach, not least because of the problem of definition. Certainly the correct definition for the purpose of HIV transmission is not someone who fits the popular image of an addict who is dependent on repeated injections of opiates at any cost. Since HIV infection can probably be transmitted by a single parenteral exposure, as we have seen from Dr Galbraith's data, the population at risk must be considered to be *"anybody who has shared injecting equipment even once".* Even occasional or experimental use is a risk. Neither can we limit the definition to users of opiates since almost any drug may be injected. This means that estimates of the drug-using population which only include those who are regularly injecting opiates will seriously underestimate the population at risk of needle-borne HIV infection.

What do we know about the size of the drug using population in Scotland? Estimates have been made as a result of two studies supported by the Standing Committee on Drug Abuse in Glasgow and Edinburgh in 1983 and 1985 respectively. These studies suggested that there were 4,300 in Glasgow and 2,000 in Edinburgh, on the basis of a multiple indicator system along the lines developed by Hartnoll[2] in London. Additionally, our colleagues in Tayside have estimated that there are perhaps a further 1,000 drug users in that region. The evidence that was presented to the Scottish Committee on HIV Infection and Intravenous Drug Misuse (SCHIIDM) was that 80% to 90% of these individuals probably injected heroin at some time. Furthermore it was estimated that there might be several thousand individuals in addition who are injecting drugs other than opiates, so our estimate, or perhaps we should more honestly call it a *guess*, was of a possible 8,000 injecting drug misusers out of the Scottish population of approximately 5 million. I think it is important to emphasise that the injection of drugs appears to be particularly common in Scotland and it seems that intensive sharing of needles was, certainly for a time, a special problem in Edinburgh and Tayside. This pattern of drug taking seems to be similar to that found in some parts of Europe and in some parts of the United States but the opinion of drug workers in England and Wales is that injection is much less common and a much higher proportion of people takes opiates by inhalation.

What proportion of Scottish drug misusers is infected with HIV? Data from several different types of study are shown in Table 2. The problem of

Table 2

Studies in Scotland recording the proportion of drug-abusers found to be HIV seropositive.

	N	% Pos		
Glasgow	606	4.5	– Laboratory	FOLLETT ET AL 1986
Tayside	129	39	identified	SMALL R G 1986 (P.C.)
			drug misusers	
Edinburgh	106	38	samples	PEUTHERER ET AL 1985
Edinburgh	164	41	– Drug misusers	ROBERTSON ET AL 1986
			attending a	
			general practice	
Edinburgh	94	54	– Drug misusers	BRETTLE ET AL 1986
			attending a	
			self referral	
			clinic for testing	

interpretation is really one of data acquisition — who gets tested and why. The first three studies listed are laboratory-based and the initial data from Glasgow, Tayside and Edinburgh depend on a decision made *by the laboratories* about which samples to test, on the basis of information given on the request form. For example, the first Edinburgh study in Table 2 was a retrospective study[1] on stored serum samples which had been submitted from one teaching hospital for hepatitis testing. They were selected because the request form said "? drug abuser".

The data of Robertson[3] and his colleagues were obtained by testing well characterised patients attending a general practice in an area of Edinburgh where drug abuse is prevalent. The method of Brettle[4] and colleagues involved individuals who were attending voluntarily, as self-referred clients, a clinic specifically set up for HIV testing of drug misusers. These individuals were pre-counselled before testing on the basis of full consent.

From all these reports it seems clear that the drug-using population in the South-East part of Scotland does have a much higher HIV-antibody prevalence than in the UK overall. These very different methods of selecting people for HIV testing obviously do give us problems in comparing the data from each study and even more so in using the findings to make an estimate of the true prevalence across the entire drug-injecting population. We also cannot measure the extent of double reporting as drug users tend to use multiple names.

For all these reasons it is very difficult to use the data available to derive an estimate of the total number of infected drug misusers in Scotland. The Scottish Committee (SCHIIDM) attempted a simple estimate based on the figures which I have given already and arrived at a figure for mid-1986 of about 1,800 HIV-infected drug misusers in Scotland. It is interesting to compare that with the current data in Table 3 which has been assembled by Dr Reid and his colleagues in the CD(S)U based on all the reports received from laboratories. The total of 611 drug misusers who are *already known* to

Table 3

Data from the CD(S)U showing the age-distribution of drug-abusers who were HIV antibody positive in Scotland from August 1983 to December 1986.

Age	Male	Female	NS	Total	(%)
0–4	4	4	—	11	
5–9	—	—	—	—	
10–14	—	—	—	—	
15–19	64	38	—	102	16.5
20–24	166	94	3	263	42.5
25–29	91	55	1	147	23.8
30–34	45	17	1	63	10.2
35–39	18	6		24	3.9
40–44	1	—		1	0.2

be positive in Scotland seems to me to fit reasonably well the sort of estimate we reached.

The assembled data from Scotland illustrate the very high proportion of all known infected people who are drug misusers and the very marked predominance of HIV infected drug misusers in some parts of the country — something like 75% of them all in the East which represents only about one third of the population. This appears to be reflected in the prevalence of HIV positivity in blood donors. In the East of Scotland, about 1 blood donor in 9,000 is HIV antibody positive. This is about five times the prevalence throughout the whole UK which is about 1 in 55,000. The excess in the East of Scotland population seems to be almost entirely due to people who have a history of drug abuse.

The evolution of the epidemic in the Scottish drug misusers seems to have followed the pattern which has been reported from several studies in Italy, although perhaps running a few years behind. The first infection appeared late in 1983 and there are several sets of data which confirm that as the starting point. A very rapid spread followed, at least in the drug users of the general practice study, so that within 18 months to two years upwards of 50% of this population had become infected.

Since then in that particular general practice population, it has been suggested that there is evidence that those who started drug use after 1983 may be showing a somewhat lower rate of new HIV infection (Figure 1). However, the data from testing of drug misusers coming to the Edinburgh Royal Infirmary (Table 4) showed a consistent positivity and there appears to be a similar situation in Dundee[5] (Table 5). No-one was positive before the end of 1983 but since then among newly tested individuals there has been quite a high proportion of antibody positives. There have been suggestions recently that the AIDS epidemic in Edinburgh is on the wane, but at present this seems unduly optimistic.

One factor which may be important in determining spread amongst drug misusers, is the apparent epidemic nature of injecting drug misuse itself.

Figure 1

The cumulative number of first positive HIV antibody test results among 83
intravenous drug abusers, by quarters (from Robertson et al 1986).

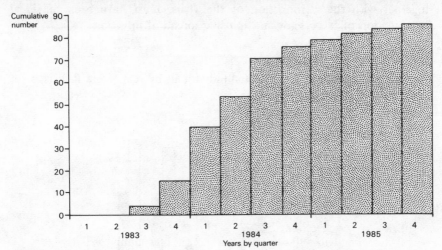

Table 4

The results of first-time HIV antibody tests on drug-abusers attending the
Edinburgh Royal Infirmary (from Peutherer JF).

	N	Positive (%)
1983	124	23(14)
1984	205	80(39)
1985	178	50(28)
1986 (Part)	178	35(20)

Table 5

The results of HIV antibody tests on drug-abusers in Tayside from June
1982 to July 1986 (from Urquhart et al 1987).

	No. Tested	No. +	% +
1982 June—Dec	20	0	0
1983 Jan—June	20	0	0
July—Dec	3	0	0
1984 Jan—June	21	10	48
July—Dec	34	16	47
1985 Jan—June	27	19	70
July*—Dec	66	40	61
1986 Jan—June	162	53	33
July	18	6	33

*July 1985 onwards—Prospective testing carried out

Brian McClelland   *83*

Figure 2 (from the general practice study) shows the apparent surge in the number of new heroin users which coincided with the first appearance of HIV. Whatever the reason for its occurrence, this outbreak of injecting, together with the introduction of the virus, must have been the ideal combination of factors for an explosive spread of infection.

Figure 2
New heroin users and HIV infected individuals by year (from Robertson et al 1986).

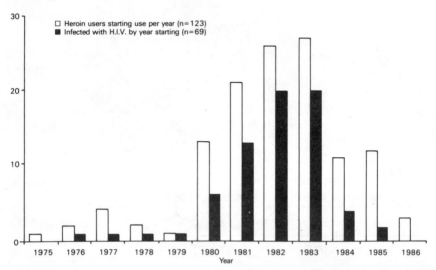

What have we learned so far from the Scottish epidemic about the spread of HIV from drug misusers to infants and to heterosexual partners who claim that they do not inject drugs? Dr Jacqueline Mok and her colleagues in Edinburgh had up to March 1987 identified 26 infants born to HIV positive mothers infected as a result of drug abuse. Of these babies, 22 have been followed up for at least 3 months and at that stage they were all, as you would expect, still seropositive. Of 20 followed up for 6 months, one had become negative, of 10 followed up for 12 months only one remained positive and this infant was symptomatic. These data are fairly representative of the European collaborative study in which three quarters of the infants enrolled had no detectable serum antibodies by one year[6]. So the suggestion from this may be that the vertical transmission from a drug-abusing mother to her baby is not all that efficient. An alternative and so far unresolved possibility is that these babies are infected but are unable to make antibodies, a suggestion that must be probed very carefully.

The other question is that of heterosexual spread as virtually all the infected drug misusers are in the reproductively active years and there is data that this group is certainly no less fertile than comparable non-drug users of similar age and social class. Heterosexual transmission is the subject of a study involving colleagues in Edinburgh, Dr Brettle and Dr Robertson, in collaboration with Professor Adler and his colleagues here. Preliminary information has been provided by Dr Brettle on 40 couples attending a self-referral screening clinic where the index case is an HIV positive drug misuser and where the heterosexual partner reports no drug injection. Of these 40 heterosexual partners who claim not to be injecting, 7 were HIV positive at first attendance and 33 were negative and have remained negative over the follow up period of up to 3 years. Thus no seroconversions have been observed during the follow up period in any of the heterosexual partners. I do not know how much reassurance one should take from this apparently low rate of transmission but we certainly need a great deal more information. This is however a very difficult group to follow up.

Finally, I think it is relevant to mention very briefly the problems that are arising in Scotland as a result of the type of policy needed to study and to control the spread of HIV related to drug abuse and the concern that these policies may appear to be condoning drug abuse. The view quite clearly expressed in the Report of the Scottish Committee (SCHIIDM)[7] was that priority should be given to the problems of containing HIV infection but not surprisingly this has been robustly opposed by a number of groups.

Despite all the useful epidemiological work that is going on, we have some immense problems in establishing reliable epidemiological information about the numbers and behaviour of drug misusers and the factors determining spread of HIV infection to their sexual partners, infants and other contacts. We will have to resolve major problems of public and professional attitudes to these issues if we are to be able to monitor the epidemic effectively and to execute and evaluate the intervention that which will be necessary to contain it.

Acknowledgement
I wish to acknowledge the generous help of Dr JF Peutherer, Dr RP Brettle, Dr Jacqueline Mok and Dr JR Robertson who permitted the use of unpublished data in this presentation. The self-referral screening clinic at the City Hospital, Edinburgh was initiated with the support of a grant from the Chief Scientist's Office, Scottish Home & Health Department.

References

1. *Peutherer JF, Edmond E, Simmonds P, Dickson JD and Bath GE*
   HTLV–III antibody in Edinburgh drug addicts
   Lancet 1985; **ii**; 1129–1130

2. *Hartnoll R et al*
   Estimating the prevalence of opioid dependence
   Lancet 1985; **i**; 203–205

3. *Robertson JR, Bucknall ABV, Welsby PD et al*
   Epidemic of AIDS-related virus (HTLV–III/LAV) infection among intravenous drug abusers
   British Medical Journal 1986; **292**; 527–529

4. *Brettle RP, Bisset K, Burns, S, Davidson J et al*
Human immunodeficiency virus and drug misuse: the Edinburgh experience
British Medical Journal 1987; **295**; 421−424

5. *Urquhart GED, Scott SS, Wooldridge E et al*
Human immunodeficiency virus (HIV) in intravenous drug abusers in Tayside
Communicable Diseases (Scotland) Reports 1987; **9**; 5−10

6. *Mok JQ, Giaquinto C, De Rossi A et al*
Infants born to mothers seropositive for human immunodeficiency virus: preliminary findings from a multicentre European study
Lancet 1987; **i**; 1164−1168

7. *Scottish Committee on HIV Infection and Intravenous Drug Misuse*
Report on HIV infection in Scotland
Scottish Home & Health Department 1986

Questions

Question
Are the babies of HIV positive mothers nursed by the mothers? Do you have information on the continuing relationship between the baby and the mother?

Dr McClelland
The majority of them are being looked after by their mothers but advice is given not to breast feed.

Question
But some of them may have breast fed before this advice.

Dr McClelland
I do not think one could exclude breast feeding completely in all cases.

Question
And do you have information on the sexual behaviour of this population? Is it different because they are drug abusers, in the frequency of intercourse for example?

Dr McClelland
No. There is published evidence from Dr Roy Robertson, the general practitioner who is looking after a group of these people, expressed in terms of their fertility, that they are if anything rather more fertile than a comparable group of non-drug using people.

Professor Anderson

I am very interested indeed in your observations about the children and your reference to the large collaborative study in Europe. Antibody decay in that study seemed to be of the same order as antibody decay for any viral infection, a half-life of the order of six months. Have you looked at these children with RNA or DNA probes to see whether they are virus positive?

Dr McClelland

That was the point I was making: all we have at the moment about these children is their antibody status. Furthermore we have only IgG antibody data, we do not even know if they have IgM. There is evidence, as I am sure you know, that there may be a higher proportion of young children than of adults who have infection without persisting antibody. The only point I can add is that the children who have persisted beyond a year with antibody, are clinically unwell.

Sir Donald Acheson

You showed a slide which I did not understand about first heroin use which suggested that there had recently been a decline in people reporting first heroin use. What is intravenous use and how was it ascertained? It seemed so encouraging I would just like a little more information.

Dr McClelland

The population was ascertained from the general practice study of Dr Robertson and so they are reasonably well known about. It was first injection that the study attempted to ascertain from patients. I am not quite sure how to interpret the data because there may be an elapsed time phenomenon, but it does appear as a simple observation that the frequency with which antibody is found is less in the group who started injecting more recently.

Dr Peterman

Of the 33 couples in which one partner remained uninfected, how many are taking precautions to avoid transmission?

Dr McClelland

I cannot give an authoritative answer on that because they are not my patients. They have all been given careful and comprehensive advice on both male and female barrier precautions and the use of spermicides. There is however some doubt how reliably they comply as there is with most groups of people. I cannot give you a meaningful answer.

Dr Peterman

I think we can all sit around and talk about what types of intervention need to be done but until someone looks at how successful we are at changing behaviour, we are not making much progress.

Dr McClelland
One observation that impressed me very much was from Dr Peter Levine who is responsible for a large group of haemophiliacs who had been counselled extremely carefully about the use of barrier contraceptive methods. He went back and interviewed them again after a few months and an alarmingly high proportion even of that very motivated group had given up such methods for a whole variety of different reasons.

Dr Peterman
I recently found out that a group of haemophiliacs in the United States had been advised not to have the antibody test so I think there is a lot of work that needs to be done in that group in the US.

Paper 10

Dr Marian McEvoy
Communicable Diseases Surveillance Centre
Public Health Laboratory Service, England & Wales

Homosexual activity data in the United Kingdom

It is important to remember that the word homosexual derives from Greek not from Latin as is often mistakenly supposed. Therefore the term emphasises the sameness of the individuals involved in a sexual relationship and not necessarily a relationship between two men. This talk concerns work which has been conducted on the behaviour of men who have engaged in sexual activity with other men.

Kinsey, who in 1948 published a study[1] of the sexual behaviour of 12,000 men in the United States of America, was perhaps the most well known researcher on this subject. He is often misquoted as having stated that 10% of the male population was homosexual but in fact his conclusion was that 10% of males are more or less exclusively homosexual for at least 3 years between the ages of 16 and 55. In fact he discovered that up to 50% of the men in his sample had had homosexual experience at some stage in their lives.

Now it is a fundamental of taxonomy that nature only rarely deals with discrete categories and Kinsey described a homosexual/heterosexual rating scaled from 0 to 6 which is based on psychological reactions and overt experiences. Scale 0 is exclusively heterosexual and scale 6 is exclusively homosexual but he stressed that an individual's rating changed at different stages throughout his life. Relatively little has been published about male homosexual practices in the United Kingdom. The work of Havelock Ellis is frequently quoted. In 1936 he estimated that between 2% and 5% of the population was homosexual but his estimate was based on extrapolation from Hirschfield's calculations for Germany published in 1920.

The definition of homosexuality is extremely important: if we take the various percentages that Kinsey described and apply them to the UK population, a range of values for this denominator of male homosexuals can be obtained from 1.1 to 12.5 million. Kinsey himself stated that satisfactory prevalence figures on the homosexual cannot be obtained by any techniques short of a carefully planned population survey. In fact if we want to do this for the population with 1% accuracy and 95% significance, we would need a sample of 10,000 and then we would be constrained by non-responders.

Recently the results of several surveys of patients attending genito-urinary medicine clinics have been presented, for example those of Whittaker (personal communication). These were small descriptive surveys concerned with the collection of socio-demographic data and the frequency of various sexual practices.

In 1984, a nationwide postal questionnaire survey was conducted by McManus and McEvoy[2] at Kings College Hospital in collaboration with the PHLS Communicable Disease Surveillance Centre. This was a purely descriptive study which was presented at the first international conference on AIDS in Atlanta in 1985. The study was designed at a very early state of the outbreak of HIV infection, before much of the present knowledge about transmission was acquired and long before mathematical modelling began. Therefore many of the points raised this morning cannot really be addressed by the results. Obviously currently designed questionnaires would be very different from those which we distributed but this was intended as a preliminary study and the questionnaires were distributed in homosexual bars, through gay magazines and gay clubs.

The aims were to describe male homosexual behaviour in the United Kingdom, to determine the sexual practices prevalent in the study group and to determine whether there were any differences in the practice of residents in London and elsewhere.

There were 1,292 responders from all regions of the United Kingdom. Altogether 40% were residents of London and 58% were from elsewhere. The age range of responders was from 18 to 70 years and about three quarters were between 20 and 39 years so it was a relatively young group. Approximately 85% placed themselves at 5 to 6 on the Kinsey scale. We did ask a question about marital status but it may not be really relevant in this type of study because it is probable that a proportion of the marriages would have been marriages of convenience. However 2% stated that they were currently involved in sexual activity with females. More than three quarters of the responders were in managerial or in skilled occupations. Altogether 15% of Londoners and 25% of those from elsewhere said they were involved in relationships with one regular male sex partner, and these relationships had endured for periods between one month and 41 years.

Although no question on the rate of exchange of partners was included, subjects were asked about the number of male partners in the previous year and this ranged from 0 to more than 500. Half had between 6 and 50 partners in the previous year but residents of London had significantly more partners. We asked about partners in a lifetime and approximately three-quarters had between 6 and 500 lifetime partners, but again Londoners had significantly more, one London man stating that he had had more than 5,000 sexual partners in his lifetime.

About 455 responders practised either receptive or insertive anal intercourse with their partners more than half the time. Around 8% were never involved in any type of anal intercourse and it was evident from the comments of the responders that activity varied with different partners, for example, someone might be receptive with a regular partner but insertive with a casual one. Very few stated that they had engaged in less well known activities such as brachio-proctic eroticism or fisting, lindinism or water sports, or coprophilia also known as scat. Residents of London were much more likely to have had previous histories of sexually transmitted diseases than those from elsewhere.

Whilst the inevitable biases in the sample were recognised, it was concluded that this type of approach was acceptable and had engendered a great deal of interest and co-operation from the gay community. London responders seemed to be more sexually active than those from elsewhere but less so than those in recent studies conducted in the United States of America. For example Bell and Weinberg[3] described higher numbers of sexual partners and higher percentages taking part in fisting etc. Unfortunately we were unable to obtain further information from the 2% who had both male and female partners and therefore we were unable to add to the conclusions of Humphries[4] who in 1970 conducted a study of cottaging, that is homosexual men who engage in sexual activities in public lavatories.

It is often supposed that men who engage in these activities might include a covert group of married men. Humphries found that such men engage largely in masturbation and oral sex with their male partners in the public lavatories and therefore they would be unlikely to play a significant role in spreading infection to their female partners. Unfortunately we are unable to add to this evidence either.

Currently there are two large surveys of male homosexual behaviour in the United Kingdom which are being co-ordinated by the Medical Research Council in order to eliminate duplication and to ensure comparability of results. The two groups are employing similar methodologies. Fitzpatrick's study will commence shortly and will concern 600 to 700 persons in five centres. About 25% of these subjects are drawn from clinics and he is going to monitor behaviour and health attitudes. Professor Coxon has a national study which will involve 750 men from 8 centres and in addition samples will be collected for serology.

Professor Coxon kindly made available the results of his pilot study. The sampling design is based on the age and type of relationship and the types are similar to those described by Bell and Weinberg: open coupled, closed coupled, functional, dysfunctional and asexual. The contacting of respondents in Professor Coxon's study proceeded initially by a variety of methods but chiefly by locating individuals known to be in one of the cells of the design. These were then asked to nominate others having the same characteristics but who were more covert than themselves, a technique known as snowball sampling.

In their pilot study, Coxon and Davies interviewed 24 men and took a sexual behaviour inventory concerning 34 sexual practices in different types of relationship and a detailed diary of sexual activity during the previous week. All subjects were then interviewed again after keeping a sexual diary for one month. Their preliminary findings were that the sexual behaviour of an individual varies extensively according to the regular partner or partners involved and whether it is a casual relationship. The sequence of sexual acts is usually individually stable and predictable but extensive differences occur between subjects. There was high initial resistance to using condoms but Coxon now feels that the situation is changing, judging from the observations in the main study, as the pilot study was conducted some time ago before the Government health education campaign.

So in conclusion, we might say that much more accurate information is needed about homosexual behaviour, in particular, that which is likely to spread infection with HIV. Also we need to provide the information that is required for modelling and prediction. It is extremely important that the extent and the acceptability of changing behaviour continues to be assessed.

References

1. *Kinsey AC, Pomeroy WB and Martin CE*
   Sexual behaviour in the human male
   Philadelphia 1948: WB Saunders

2. *McManus TJ and McEvoy MB*
   Some aspects of male homosexual behaviour in the UK
   British Journal of Sexual Medicine 1987; **14(4)**; 110-118

3. *Bell AP and Weinberg MS*
   Homosexualities: a study of diversities between men and women
   London 1979: Mitchell Beazley

4. *Humphries RA*
   The Tea Room Trade: impersonal sex in public places
   Chicago 1970: Aldvic

Questions and General Discussion

Professor Anderson
I enjoyed very much this very interesting paper. In relation to the Fitzpatrick and Coxon studies, have they been designed so that both rate of partner change and duration of the different partners are determined. The sort of question that will be asked is how many partners in the last month, 2 months, 6 month, 1 year, 5 years etc so that we can assess how the mean and variance of these distributions change. In particular the lumping of categories in the high partner change zone has to be very carefully examined because that could alter the variance substantially.

Dr McEvoy
Yes indeed, I have only been able to look at Professor Coxon's protocol but those questions would certainly be asked and in a quantitative way.

Professor Knox
I heard Professor Coxon presenting his results just recently. It is based on sexual diaries and each event and each act is exhaustively recorded and then coded for entry on the computer. The main problem is recording it in a way which the coder can understand and his wife cannot if she finds it in with his socks.

Question

You made some comparisons between the United Kingdom and the United States in the prevalence of certain homosexual habits. Could you tell us a little bit more about that because it is rather a key issue in predicting what is going to happen.

Dr McEvoy

It may not be entirely valid to make those comparisons here, though. The Bell and Weinberg study was conducted in San Francisco and so we are comparing results from that with our study. They certainly found that their responders had higher numbers of sexual partners both in the lifetime and in the previous year. They also found that a higher number of those they interviewed admitted to engaging in some more bizarre practices. We find a very low percentage of those. Our studies were really conducted in different ways, in particular ours was distributed in a magazine that was in public circulation. Now this may have inhibited some of our responders from giving us precise information about these practices, there is a suggestion that the practices are different but by no means could one be conclusive about this.

Question

Could I raise a question with you? I remember talking to Dr McManus about the possibility of combining serology with your study. Was that possible in the end?

Dr McEvoy

After our preliminary study was undertaken, Dr McManus subsequently incorporated his study in that of Professor Coxon which I believe does include some sero-epidemiology.

Question

It does seem to be rather important I think, the real crunch point, we are not primarily interested in homosexual behaviour but in the spread of infection. Does all this relate or can it be related to the transmission of an infectious agent. We did talk about the possibility of looking at other infections besides HIV. I hope that will be possible as well.

Dr JWG Smith

I remember looking at the protocols and being concerned that the size of the sample might not be large enough to be able to support serological findings and to get a prospective estimate of the risk factors from homosexual activity. I am wondering whether there has been any further assessment whether you will secure enough seroconversions in the study population to relate this to sexual activities.

Dr McEvoy

I do not know if there have been further developments. I gather that the study population was calculated as 750 as a minimum required but Coxon will be recruiting rather more than this, perhaps 1,000 or more.

Question

Can I ask our American colleagues if there are any studies which relate behaviour to acquisition of infection rather than the studies we know about in connection with risk of disease?

Question

There are a couple of studies that have recently been published which report incidence in people with varying behaviours. There is a very high correlation with anal receptive intercourse.

Question

The Winkelstein study is really the best one of that character simply because it looked at a group that was not just high risk. There is a much broader stratification of the sample and the evidence from that about rate of partner change and the probability of being seropositive in 1986 is extremely good.

Dr JWG Smith

I think it is quite an important study in the sense that the estimate of the risk of different sexual practices has come from retrospective studies of behaviour, such as the one Philip Mortimer has been involved with. But the chances of estimating it prospectively, even amongst the homosexual population, is very small because the seroconversion rate is quite low from year to year and I do not think that we should expect that sort of result to come from only 700 people.

Question

I suppose it would depend partly also in what area it was done. Looking at different centres, in some the frequency of seropositivity is much higher than in others, though I agree that wherever you go the rate of seroconversion is likely to be low.

Professor Adler

The rate of seroconversion is slowing down in homosexual men because thay have taken the message about safe sex. Therefore I think you are quite right in saying that it is prospectively unlikely that you will pick anything up in terms of particular sexual practices in relation to seroconversion rates. In fact most of them are not engaging in those dangerous practices any more.

Dr Meade Morgan

I would disagree with that in some ways. In Boston we have a cohort where we have identified more or less monogamous homosexual couples. In several couples enrolled in the study we have identified one man who is seropositive for HIV while the other man is negative. They have been counselled about safe sexual practice but many of them have refused to use those methods feeling that they must be immune if they already have the infection. So there is this kind of denial among at least certain people in the sexual community.

Professor Adler

I accept that but there are going to be people who do not take the advice that they are given. In global terms, particularly in London where we are seeing most of the high risk homosexuals, there is some sort of change in behaviour if you look at it in group terms. Obviously there will be individuals who are not subscribing to safe sex behaviour.

Question

I was sent some data from the Netherlands of a prospectively collected study of a large group of homosexuals who were recruited for some other reason. That certainly showed very strong correlation of seropositivity with all the things you would expect and anal receptive practices had a higher rate. Other factors had a protective effect because they kept them off the more dangerous behaviour. There was also a strong correlation with numbers of partners. He had asked them how often contact was anonymous, in what proportion of the partners did they not exchange names etc. The higher the anonymity again the higher the risk of transmission so this did seem to conform and the numbers were quite considerable.

Question

Can I ask you another question which perhaps you could answer jointly with Spence Galbraith. Have you evidence about how the present degree of sexual activity is allowing the virus to spread geographically outside the London area where you have done most of your work? Have you related what you have found about behaviour to where the virus seems to be moving?

Dr Galbraith

We have no further information from the surveillance system than I showed. We have not connected it up with the homosexual data which Dr McEvoy has presented.

Professor Adler

I think one of the points, of course, about the data that is contained here in terms of seropositivity is that it is not necessarily representative because only PHLS laboratories are reporting it. I think that goes back to one of the very early points we made this morning, that there is an urgent need to have anonymous screening set up nationally that would give us representative samples throughout the United Kingdom of different risk groups at different levels of risk.

Professor A Glynn

May I make the point that theoretically it is not only PHLS laboratories that are reporting, all laboratories report and Dr Galbraith will confirm that a large part of our information on all diseases comes from outside the PHLS. There are of course one or two very distinguished laboratories which do not report, but I will not name them.

Dr Meade Morgan

One comment for Professor Adler with regard to anonymous testing as we had a meeting at CDC about 3 weeks ago to discuss the issue of mandatory serologic testing around the country. We discussed voluntary testing versus anonymous testing and there was a strong consensus among the public health people at the meeting that even anonymous testing might be bad in the sense that it may prevent people from attending the Sexually Transmitted Disease (STD) clinics for the treatment they need. So if you do put that type of programme in place you do need to be very careful.

Dr P Mortimer

Could I just make an observation about this problem of marriage between study of behaviour and serology? We have a lot of data now from retrospective surveys and from prospective surveys on cohorts. I am wondering more and more whether we should not look more at the other approach which is to have some sampling tool which is really based on a nationally agreed simple questionnaire. This can be administered in very many different contexts but perhaps everyone could have some input into designing it. It can be used over a period of time, not on the same clinic population but clearly on different individuals over time, and with some simple serological investigation.

The first time I heard this suggestion put forward was by Dr Emslie from the Scottish Communicable Diseases Unit at a meeting. Taken with the technological advances in testing, particularly in the ability that several groups now have to test saliva as opposed to serum, this suggests to me that we could put together something that would allow us to use this questionnaire and marry it with decent serology to study the way the epidemic is going and the impact of changes of behaviour following information campaigns etc. It is a different approach to the small cohort where there is always criticism that it is a clinic population. That is what happens in San Francisco but that sort of criticism should not happen here.

Chairman

I think you do have to define very clearly what it is you are going to look for. A high power microscope is a very valuable tool but sometimes you need to use the low power. I would not have the cohorts knocked, even if Professor Adler were not here, because they have taught us a lot about the way in which we can study the evolution of the infection in detail. I entirely agree with your point that you have a different purpose where cohort studies will not give the answers we want. I should be Chairman, not taking part in the discussion.

——————————— *End of Third Session* ———————————

Fourth Session

Chairman Sir Donald Acheson
Chief Medical Officer
Department of Health & Social Security, England

Open Discussion

Chairman

This is the opportunity for those of you who feel that you have something to say but have not had an opportunity because the rest of us have been talking so much. Please say whatever it is you want to say. Furthermore, of course, one of the objects of the meeting is for this distinguished international group of people to offer advice to those of us in the United Kingdom who are interested in this problem. I hope you will take that into account also.

But to begin with, I have asked two colleagues to say something: one is Norman Bailey and the other is Alan Glynn. First, Professor Bailey.

Professor Bailey

Thank you, Mr Chairman. I would like to make a few comments on matters that I think we have not yet covered. We have heard a great deal about the development of scientific models, long-term models that need good data to provide understanding. My prejudices are very much in favour of this kind of work which I enjoy. To settle down to this sort of task is both fun and interesting and the result may be useful in the long run. I also think a lot of work has been done on infectious diseases, on past data where the models fitted and could be made to produce good predictions. I am thinking of the work done by the Soviet Union over the period 1967 onwards which made predictions about what would happen from one city to another in the spread of influenza. The confirmation of this work by colleagues in Geneva and others in the US and in the UK, showed for example that the 1968 Hong Kong epidemic could be modelled and predictions could be made about the spread of influenza on a global basis. But this is all twenty years back.

The problem now is what do we do with a disease which is spreading currently, where we cannot wait twenty years to do good modelling. We need more discussion about the problems facing Ministers of Health. In the UK I assume that many decisions have to be made right now about various matters: health campaigns, the medical services that will be required, the numbers of beds, medical staff, availability of drugs, and so on, together with the planning of research for future developments, so as to keep abreast of what is done.

In addition to the scientifically respectable modelling efforts, there are immediate needs for benchmark figures that will enable administrators to cope with demands now as well as in the immediate years ahead. We need approximate methods which will allow us to make calculations about the likely volume of these needs, and I would suggest — this is a big subject — we need some kind of adaptive planning of the kind already done on adaptive surveillance and management in the systems field.

From what we have heard, particularly in the modelling of human behaviour, not only is human behaviour very variable but it is extremely sensitive to various kinds of assumptions and it is going to be a long time before we have a really accurate picture. The result is that we get models with large numbers of compartments in them, lots of transitions between them, and although one can make synthetic investigations to say what would happen conditionally, this does have a very large standard error attached to it. I suspect what we really need in the short run, if it can be done, is a robust model which is valid broadly for public health needs supported by careful long-term scientific work.

With regard to anxieties about spread to the heterosexual population, since this spread has already started (although the numbers are not very large), we can consider that the heterosexual side of the epidemic has already been triggered. It may be the influence of drug-takers, bisexuals, or prostitutes but this is not now quite as important as it would otherwise be because the infection now has a life of its own in the main risk groups. We should certainly look at the mathematical aspects of that to see if we can produce some valid figures in the short run.

That is all I really wish to say. There are a number of technical points that I have already discussed with individuals but I think my main view relates to what the Department of Health needs right now and what kind of robust models could be developed quickly — maybe they already exist — in order to aid ongoing decision-making.

Chairman
Thank you very much for that practical approach. Does anyone want to reflect on that?

Professor Anderson
I think I agree in part with Norman Bailey about the need for some guidance. The statistical estimates extrapolating from an exponential curve will provide us with something for the coming year or so. However, if we are happy with very wide confidence limits and the epidemiologists and virologists are prepared to assume an incubation period as of the order of 8 years with further assumptions about whether people are infectious throughout this period, then crude bench mark figures could be provided now, particularly as we have data on the rising incidence.

And also, we could adapt such very simple crude models to incorporate the apparent changes in sexual behaviour from the data on the decline in incidence of gonorrhoea in homosexuals, so we could take account of the trend in sexual habits.

Chairman
But I feel sure we would need data at least as good as you would normally publish in the scientific literature.

Dr Tyrrell
On these lines, it has occured to me that one might try and take the epidemic apart. If we can get a reasonable estimate of the number of seropositives now existing and work from their rate of becoming sick, at least we could get an interim estimate of the total number of cases that may occur and when they may occur. This separates what to me is a rather more tricky question, that of working out how the virus will spread. This depends on what people will be doing and thinking in a few years time and such results

must be more than usually indeterminate. Even if we knew all the facts now and people went on behaving as they are now, it would still be very difficult to predict the epidemic. It is intrinsically impossible, I think, to be sure what will be happening in the way of transmission in the coming five years or so.

I think we have to live with this but I must say that short-term predictions and other imperfect measures may nevertheless be helpful, accessible and sufficiently accurate.

Dr JWG Smith

Michael Healy referred to Russian work on the epidemiology of influenza, they of course have a great advantage in that they can work out very precisely the transfer of people between centres during the winter because they are separated by snows and the transport is entirely by aeroplane and by train.

In the AIDS field, we are in quite a different ball game, particularly in Western Europe where contact between the infected and the uninfected is far more free and almost uncontrollable. Thus, unlike the Russians with their influenza, we will have to accept wide confidence limits in forecasting AIDS.

Professor Knox

Could I comment on two general methods of working because I have been used to working in one way and watching other people work in the other way. If we have to make a decision and have to make a prediction, which is the public health position, then we must use models. There is no doubt about that. They may be explicit models, they may be diagrammatic models, or they may be mental models, but their use is the only way to predict the future.

The way I have worked in this and in other fields is to start with something crude and then gradually improve its resolution and its accuracy. Partly this is helped as data comes along but partly it is the modeller's resolve. Firstly we introduce age, then time, and so on. The model gradually becomes more complex, the data gradually get better and the predictions, one hopes, gradually improve as well. That is one way of working.

The other way, and I am not accusing anyone of doing this, starts with collection of every detail and no predictions are made until every detail is shown on paper with dozens of loops and compartments. Carried to its absurd extreme, this never provides an answer during anybody's lifetime!

I think we must work in both directions. We have no choice in this situation as we want a result quickly. If it has to be nasty, then it has to be nasty and we will get better as we go on. That is the way I prefer to work.

Dr Mann

It is worth coming back to a basic question: if we do not know how many people in any population are infected and who they are, then how can we proceed? I think it is a fundamental question for a chronic communicable disease like AIDS. I realise that there are ethical and legal problems with the development of this information, but having this information will allow us to say a great deal. The information that has been developed from a variety of cohort studies gives a relatively clear idea of where we are going and where we are right now. It will not tell you how many people will be infected next year — that is another question — but I think this is a key question and it is worth addressing the difficult issues involved to try to obtain that information.

Dr Mortimer

Could I make a comment about prediction in the UK which echoes what Dr Tyrrell was saying. If we consider only what may happen up to the end of this decade, we are looking at a group of potential AIDS cases almost all of whom are already infected with the virus. What happens in the 1990s concerns quite largely a group of people who have yet to be infected. With regard to short-term prediction, that which involves this decade only, the empiricists win and the modellers do not have anything like so much to contribute.

There seem two ways in which we can look at short-term prediction. Extrapolation, as Roy Anderson says, will work for a year, eighteen months or perhaps two years and tell us something. The experience we have seen in the United States has many demographic similarities. If we allow that we are perhaps three years behind and our population is something like a quarter of what it is in the United States, then we come up with a series of figures for AIDS in the UK which do in fact quite closely parallel what was happening in the United States three years ago. So there are two very empirical ways of thinking what might happen in the next two or three years in the United Kingdom.

Both of them, looking at how those approaches have developed, tend to state the worst case the the real case that we are now observing is something rather less than that. Perhaps the worst case is what we need and not the more optimistic one which may mislead on policy formation.

The way in which modellers might help us in the short-term is to produce a better estimate of the existing number of seropositives as it is quite clear that the cases of AIDS in the next two or three years are going to be drawn from that population of seropositives. Sadly at the moment there is so much duplication, so much under-reporting, that we can only guess at seropositives at the moment.

Dr Aron

The National Cancer Institute have developed methods which I have been discussing with Roy Anderson and he thinks they have some degree of bias, they use an approach working off reported AIDS cases with an assumption about the incubation period. Each method has its own biases but this in combination with some measure of seropositivity, which is going to have its own set of problems, might I think be able to come up with some confident estimates of the next few years.

Professor A Glynn

I was very interested to hear Roy Anderson say this morning that he thought the most important need at the moment was that the model should be tested against the facts. Clearly that puts all the virologists and epidemiologists on their mettle to produce some facts they may be used for testing. I think that is right because all the models have used well known basic epidemiological principles and have converted them algebraically into some formulae which hopefully will yield predictions when the constants are available. At the moment they cannot predict because we do not have the constants to put in, but I think we should be able to produce the constants soon. I would like to stress once again how important it is, whatever the drawbacks, that primarily this should be data on HIV seropositivity more than AIDS cases, because the cases are a reflection of what happened a few years ago, whereas we really want to know what is happening now in terms of people being infected.

Spence Galbraith showed very clearly how the surveillance works, both of cases and of antibody-positive people. I think these systems of surveillance have to continue, and have to be refined and extended, but they have their limitations and we will not get enough data from them without enormous resource input. We do need to look more carefully at how we can mount a survey directed at answering specific questions like the common one at the moment: how far has infection spread into the heterosexual community?

There are, as you know, some surveys going on at the Middlesex Hospital and the PHLS designed to do that, but it will take a little time because it looks as if the penetration into the heterosexual community is very slight at the moment. It is only just reaching the limits of measurement and the slight variations that people look at are really noise fluctuations at a very low level. Of course, what we want to do is to pick it up before it reaches a really significant level.

One of the surveys is that based on STD clinics which has started relatively recently. In the 1985 figures, where very few people were surveyed, there were only 146 heterosexual women looked at and none of those was seropositive. For 1986 we only have data for the first three-quarters of the year and of about 600 women tested none was positive either. This present year the study has expanded and there should be very many more women tested so it will be interesting to see when we get the first seropositive.

The other encouragement following the Government's information programme of the last few months, is that the number of tests carried out has increased considerably. Some laboratories are doing double or triple what they were and creaking under the strain because they are not just dealing with extra HIV tests — patients attending STD clinics also generate laboratory requests for chlamydia, syphilis, and other serology so the work-load shoots up.

It is very interesting that the total number of seropositives has remained roughly the same although the total number of HIV tests has shot up, so the Government's information programme has not uncovered some hidden well of infected people. There are large numbers who think they are at risk and have come to be tested, but it is very encouraging that the number found seropositive has remained much the same as before.

Dr Philip Mortimer made a plea for distributed testing round the country, which I think has a real place together with more directed surveys. He also mentioned the technology of saliva testing which he has done a lot to develop. It is going to be a very difficult public relations exercise to persuade people that they do not get AIDS from saliva despite the fact that we can detect the presence of the virus from tests upon saliva.

I do not wish to get into the argument about the ethics of anonymous testing because I do not think this is the place, but there is the traditional public health dilemma that there are still those, including medical people, who write to the papers saying: "Why are we making all this fuss about AIDS? There are only 700!". If we do our job properly there may be little increase on the present 30,000 or so seropositives and they will say: "What was all the fuss about?" If we do not do it properly, of course, the result will be awful.

Chairman
Who else would like to say something? Particularly those who have not had an opportunity.

Dr Johan Giesecke
I talked to Dr McClelland about our testing in Sweden of pregnant women. This was started six months ago and has been very successful. We started in the southern half of Stockholm, testing all pregnant women who came to the antenatal clinic, whether for an abortion or to have their child. It has been very well received by these women and 99% have accepted the test. Known drug addicts are taken out of this cohort and so far 4,000 women have been tested and of which two were seropositive — one of them was born in Africa and the other one was probably infected elsewhere. That is one of the screening procedures and it has been working very well.

The second is just starting now at the Stockholm Jail where all the drug addicts are tested if they wish. The police report that almost all intravenous drug addicts pass through the jail over a two-year period, that is the best way to pick them up!

The third method is in a couple of hospitals where we have tested all blood samples that come to the laboratory in one day. The samples are unidentified and pooled. We will repeat that every half year to determine the prevalence of seropositivity of those in the hospital.

Chairman
Could I ask in clarification whether or not the individuals in these groups are asked for their consent?

Dr Johan Giesecke
Yes, the pregnant women and the prisoners are asked to consent to the tests. The third group is really for occupational health considerations of the staff in the clinical chemistry laboratory of the hospital. They want to know how many of the blood samples they get are infected, so that is done anonymously. Although the subjects do not know their blood samples are being tested, there is no way of linking the results to the individuals afterwards.

Question

Do you know the proportion of drug addicts in the prison?

Dr Johan Giesecke

No, the prison study started on 1 January 1987 and we have around 10% drug addicts but they were all known beforehand and the seropositives we found so far were all previously tested elsewhere.

Dr McClelland

I have a question for Dr Mann who mentioned the differences between countries. The data that I presented and the data of Spence Galbraith about the UK show that we have a country within a country epidemiologically at the moment. In Edinburgh the epidemiology of seropositivity is completely different from the rest of the UK. Even Glasgow which is just a 30-minute train ride away from Edinburgh, has still a low seroprevalence in the drug abusers.

From your global view of the problem, do you think there are important lessons for the UK in how we should approach the question of containment of what is still a localised drug-abuser epidemic?

Dr Mann

I do not think anyone has an answer yet how to control or contain an IV drug-abuser epidemic. There are strategies being used but I think these strategies are difficult to evaluate. Nor do they readily allow determination which factors may be influencing the epidemic.

Worldwide there is very little we can say other than point to the apparently obvious strategies. We have places where condom use is increasing, but where we do not yet have any idea whether infection rates are decreasing or stabilising. So I think we are still very much at the phase I described as the "early phase" where we do what we think is right on the basis of what we know about the descriptive epidemiology of the disease and the people at risk.

Chairman

Thank you. Dr Meade Morgan, we have heard a lot today about how we should improve our knowledge of the prevalence of the virus infection. Are there any lessons we can learn from the United States on this?

Dr Meade Morgan

I will be glad to tell you what our thinking is in the United States and you can decide for yourselves whether there are any lessons worth learning.

As I mentioned earlier, about three weeks ago we held a conference in Atlanta with about 500 attending from various health departments around the country. We addressed three main questions:

1. how serological screening could be done as part of the process of getting a marriage licence, as in the United States we already screen for syphilis and gonorrhoea;

2. whether all those coming to an STD clinic for treatment should be required to be screened for the AIDS virus;

3. whether all hospital admissions should be screened.

Within each of those three categories we considered possible methods of screening. For mandatory screening, how should the information be protected? Is it public information or should safeguards be placed on the data in terms of confidentiality? We also considered the role of anonymous screening purely for public health purposes. That is, there would be no way we could go back to a person and make them aware of their serological status, the idea being again that we need to try and monitor the spread of the AIDS virus.

The overwhelming consensus at the meeting was that they did not like any of these methods; they thought any screening has to be purely voluntary and that the person screened needs to know in advance that he is being screened. This was done to ensure that people would feel willing to come and use the medical facilities made available to them. This reaction surprised us at CDC. I was expecting a little more debate on the matter but there was very little.

We do have certain programmes that we are putting in place to try and monitor the spread of the virus. There are the Red Cross blood testing, the military recruits that I mentioned before, and the sentinel hospitals where we are doing anonymous screening. We had a lot of trouble getting that proposal through our internal review boards, but the feeling was that the public health benefit outweighed other ethical considerations. Perhaps my colleague Dr Tom Peterman has some thoughts on that?

Dr Peterman
I think it is important to make a distinction between screening for the benefit of the person you are testing and serologic studies which are designed to determine the prevalence in a population. There are a number of places that are doing anonymous seroprevalence studies and there are centres which treat sexually-transmitted diseases that are screening anonymously to see what the burden is in their population.

Dr P Mortimer
The information from Dr Giesecke of Sweden, that 99% of antenatal patients were willing to be screened, is very interesting and obviously conflicts with what came out of the conference in Atlanta. I have been told on several occasions that it would be unacceptable to screen in our antenatal clinics or to screen heterosexuals in genito-urinary clinics. I wonder whether the time has come to carry out a survey of the patients coming to those clinics and ask them whether or not they object to being tested, rather than expect obstetricians or other groups to represent the view of patients.

Dr McClelland
I can comment on that. We were investigating the possibility of anonymous screening in the antenatal population in Edinburgh and, as part of that

exercise, a small survey is being made at the moment to ask precisely the question that Philip Mortimer has raised. This is extremely preliminary data which I had not intended to mention but the answer that appears to be coming out is exactly what our colleagues in Sweden have discovered: that pregnant mothers offered the opportunity of some form of testing, virtually all say: "Yes please, and we want to have the result!".

Chairman
This is hardly screening. It is testing with consent, is it not?

Professor Anderson
I too was very surprised by the attitude in the Atlanta meeting about screening because the US is the one country that legislates for immunisation of young children. Quite clearly the ethical issue lying behind that asks the individual to protect himself for the benefit of the community as a whole, and in this country we have problems with that issue.

The other broader difficulty about screening is that the likely figure for seropositivity is going to be very low. If that figure becomes widely known in the press, the public's perceived risk will be: "Good! Forget about it! It does not affect me, it is so low!". The main point to get across is I think the time-scale of this characteristic of the epidemic rather than that *very* low prevalence of infection. This is something that is going to move very slowly, that education has not put across yet.

Chairman
Also, as you pointed out, there is a lot of heterogeneity.

Dr JWG Smith
One point that has not come out quite clearly is that we have been talking about the advantage mathematical modelling may give in indicating the use of resources etc. I think it also has an important preventive role as it can identify where intervention strategies are likely to be most effective. For this reason modelling is particularly important in all countries.

Dr Meade Morgan
Returning to screening for a moment, there is one other point I would like to mention. Screening programmes that are set up are going to be quite an economic burden on resources. Not only are we going to be screening but we will have to provide counselling and education both to the people that are seropositive and probably to those that are negative. If it is voluntary screening, they are probably coming in because they consider themselves at risk, for whatever reason, so not only are we running the test but we have to offer these support services and pay for them.

Professor A Glynn
There is evidence, recently published, that drug abuse has fallen over the last two years which suggests that they have taken notice of the campaigns. I wonder if there are two populations: one that is not permanent within the

normal course of events where individuals may come off drugs in a year or so, perhaps this is the group that is giving up more quickly. Then the other group, and perhaps smaller group, who are presently failing to respond. Is anything known about the history of drug abusers?

Chairman
Anyone like to answer on that one. Dr McClelland, you must be fairly well-versed in that.

Dr McClelland
At second-hand, Sir, but the answer to the question is that there is much known about the natural history of drug abusers. They are a highly heterogeneous group, ranging from those who are permanently and classically addicted to people who experiment but stop for very long periods and do not inject at all. In any population that has been looked at in Europe you will find everything between those extremes.

The other point was the one which I tried to illustrate very hastily in my talk. This was that the phenomenon of intravenous heroin use appears to be an epidemic phenomenon and that there was an epidemic in this country which started about 1980 and is now definitely declining. I think that decline probably started well before any of the current public information campaigns, so it would be inappropriate to attribute it to what has gone on in the last few months.

Professor Bailey
Perhaps I could ask a question. Since we have all been called here to discuss these matters involving clinical aspects, serology, epiodemiology, bias, statistics, modelling, public health decision-making and so on, one wonders what will happen to it all. If it is to be of any use, all this has to be integrated and there has to be some kind of action taken, presumably at the level of the DHSS. One of the points I mentioned earlier was the adaptive approach. Operational research should be carried out on an adaptive basis in which a small number of experts from different fields work together, some of them in an academic or research institution, some of them close to the decision-makers.

I was just wondering whether there are any plans to do this in order to bring together the problems and approaches we have been discussing and make sure that the academic work really is kept in line with the needs of the decision-makers.

Chairman
I can assure you that what has been said today will not be lost. The presentations, questions and discussion have been recorded and we will have them edited and published. I think there is no doubt at all that this has been an extremely good meeting. For Professor Bailey, I will personally be in touch with you about this particular point that you have mentioned.

Perhaps we can then turn to Michael Healy and ask him to attempt the impossible and have a go at summing up the main points of what we have said today.

Summing Up Professor M J R Healy
London School of Hygiene & Tropical Medicine
University of London

I take it that when the Chief Medical Officer chose me to sum up this meeting, he was looking for someone who would give an unprejudiced view, free from preconceptions. Insofar as this equates with "ignorant", I think he has made a successful choice.

The main impression that I have gained is of the extreme complexity of the AIDS forecasting problem. For a start, there seem to be three epidemics in progress with loose links between them. The main epidemic, numerically speaking, is in male homosexuals. This epidemic has been quite extensively studied in the USA and to some extent here, and we know a certain amount about it. For example, we know what types of sexual behaviour are most likely to lead to transmission of the disease, and we have a limited amount of information, in America, Europe and in our own country, on the prevalences of these types of behaviour. We do lack solid information on denominators, the sizes of the populations involved, but our state of knowledge on this epidemic is far from null.

Next comes the epidemic, linked to the first, in intravenous drug abusers. This epidemic has great geographic variability — our Edinburgh colleagues have about as much experience as anyone in the world. Here again, behavioural factors are of great importance. Even before AIDS came along, the behaviour of drug abusers had been the subject of a great deal of research, and I am sure that a lot of the results of this work are currently being fed into AIDS epidemiology.

Thirdly, we have the epidemic that frightens us all, that in the heterosexual population. The numbers potentially involved are far greater, and here we seem to know almost nothing. Nobody, as I understand it, can tell me whether such an epidemic exists or not at the present time. Some heterosexual people are becoming seropositive or manifesting the disease, but whether or not there are enough to maintain an epidemic seems quite uncertain. One main objective of public health policy should presumably be to prevent this epidemic from happening at all.

One thing that we know for certain is that we have available at the present time only one potentially effective method of prevention, which consists in education, propaganda or advice. The possibility of drug treatment is real, that of a vaccine fairly remote, but for the purpose of immediate policy, education is all that we have. This, along with one further point, makes this a strange epidemic for epidemiologists. The further point was made by Normal Bailey when he noted that this is the first major epidemic that epidemiologists have been asked to study as it occurs, rather than in the academic historical atmosphere that has tended to surround studies of infectious diseases in developed countries.

One implication of this struck me forcibly in viewing one of Professor Anderson's slides. This showed a possible predicted course of the epidemic over some 40 to 50 years, with a plotted rectangle for each year rising to a peak and falling to a plateau. Professor Anderson then pointed to the present time, just discernible at the bottom left hand end of the diagram around rectangle number 5. It seems clear that we cannot yet have the information to assess the reliability of these long term forecasting models.

The second lesson that I have learned today is summed up by George Knox when he points out that we can only cope with simplified models of reality. The problem, of course, is the extent to which simplification can safely be carried. We have heard today about two different levels of simplification. At one extreme we have what may be called empirical forecasting — put crudely, we plot the points against time and draw a line through them. Alternatively, we can attempt to model the ways in which infection spreads by setting up sets of more or less complicated differential equations.

We have been given an impressive example of empirical forecasting by Dr Meade Morgan. It is no reflection on his work if I say that it illustrates the limitations of the method. Amusingly, he quoted 67% confidence limits for his forecasts rather than the more conventional 95% limits. I am of course delighted to see someone breaking with this rather mindless contention, but I suspect that one of the reasons for doing so was that the lower 95% limit quite quickly became negative. As Professor Anderson points out, empirical forecasting is probably the best we can do for the very short term, but its level of uncertainty rapidly becomes unacceptable.

There is perhaps a bit more mileage to be got out of the empirical approach. The AIDS epidemic in this country is several years behind that in America and roughly contemporary with those in European countries. While there are substantial differences between these epidemics in certain respects, they are not wholly unrelated and it may be possible to improve the extrapolation of our own figures if we relate them in a more or less formal manner to those relating to other countries.

To go further into this picture we need to put together all our knowledge of virology and sociology so as to build up a fairly detailed picture of the way in which the infection spreads. We have heard today about several of these mathematical models, and their results have been displayed, though not always with the caution that Professor Anderson showed in concealing the scale on the y-axis. What we ask for from a model is an accurate forecast of the future. We can put into the model as much as we can of current knowledge (sparse as this may turn out to be), but the only confirmatory test we can carry out is to verify the accuracy with which the model has imitated the past. We run straight into the difficulty that I have already mentioned, that the epidemic is still at a very early stage, so that good correspondence with the past is consistent with widely different forecasts of the future, at least in a quantitative sense.

As a side-issue, it may be known that I am interested in what does and does not constitute scientific work. There is considerable pressure at all times to be as scientific as possible. Mathematical modelling of epidemics is a well-known scientific area, full of interesting problems, and the complexity of the AIDS epidemic ensures that it will supply plenty of new ones. Today has provided evidence that these problems will be actively pursued. But we are confronted as a nation with more than the problem of acquiring new knowledge that is the business of science. We also need solutions to what I call the technological problem of achieving certain pre-defined goals — here, of preventing or containing the AIDS epidemic. I hope that there will be equal enthusiasm for tackling these problems, of which forecasting is only one. We shall need both scientific and technological approaches to the worst part of all, what to do in the 1990s when I feel that at present we have very little to offer. It would be nice to be in the position of the solver of chess problems who is allowed to claim "no solution" as a correct and satisfactory answer, but I believe that Ministers of the Crown and their advisers are not permitted this escape route.

This brings me to the third lesson I have learned from today's proceedings. One reason that we are unable to forecast the epidemic in more than qualitative terms is that we have not got the necessary information. The models we have heard about contain large numbers of numerical parameters, both single numbers and whole distributions, whose values we do not possess. What are the most urgent needs in this direction?

First seems to come the frequency of infection with the HIV. This sounds simple enough, but we do not know the answer, certainly not when the population is broken down into the important subgroups. Next we need to know about varieties of sexual behaviour and the extent to which they change over time. Much of our baseline data is drawn from the Kinsey report, which relates to many years ago in a quite different society and which has in any case been heavily criticised by statisticians. Even if we had baseline information, we know little about changes in behaviour or even about ways of measuring such changes. The participants in today's meeting may not even include the people who are really expert in this field.

Although we possess a good deal of methodology relevant to these problems and to others which could be added to them, we are operating in areas which are unfamiliar to many epidemiologists. Above all, we run continually into ethical difficulties — we have to ask not about the practicability of collecting certain information, but about its acceptability. I believe that the views of the general public on these matters need deeper exploration. The opinions of pregnant women in Edinburgh and in Sweden have been briefly reported to us and may lead to greater optimism (or less pessimism) about large-scale testing than some of us might have expected.

And so, to the surprise of nobody but the dismay of some, we reach the usual conclusion of these exercises — what is needed is more research. Yet the conclusion is here very clear. We need, as a matter of urgency, new and better information about the epidemic, and as a first step a clear formulation of what that information should consist of. We need far better communication between those working on the problem. The Royal Statistical Society is planning to do something for the statisticians by holding a specialised workshop in May or June and a larger public meeting in the autumn. I believe that other workers have equally serious communication problems, with far too many people unwilling to discuss with each other what they are doing and how they are doing it. I am delighted to see Dr Dietz and our American colleagues here, to say nothing of Dr Mann from WHO, but I would be happier if the forecasting work that is going on outside this country could be put beside our own contributions, to the benefit of both.

I have tried, Sir Donald, to give some kind of bird's eye view of the forecasting situation as I have learned about it today. The risks of bird's eye views are to those standing underneath; I hope that mine has been on balance of some usefulness in drawing the proceedings to a close.

Chairman

Thank you very much, Michael Healy for a characteristically brilliant and humorous conclusion and summary of today's meeting.

Before we finish, could I just thank on your behalf those who have organised this meeting, Dr Fenton Lewis and his group who made all the arrangements and brought you all here. Thank you very much Dr. Lewis.

Many of us will be meeting again later this evening at dinner and I look forward very much to seeing you there. Thank you all very much for coming and for contibuting to this important discussion.

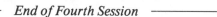 *End of Fourth Session*

Those attending

Participants

Rt Hon Norman Fowler MP   Secretary of State for Social Services

Sir Donald Acheson   Chief Medical Officer,
Department of Health & Social Security

Professor F O'Grady   Chief Scientist,
Department of Health & Social Security

Dr David Tyrrell   Chairman, Working Party on AIDS
Medical Research Council

Dr J W G Smith   Director, Public Health Laboratory Service

Professor R A Anderson   Imperial College, University of London

Dr Meade Morgan   Centers for Disease Control AIDS Unit,
Atlanta

Professor Klaus Dietz   Tübingen University

Professor H W Hethcote   Iowa University

Professor E G Knox   Birmingham University

Professor Sir David Cox   Imperial College, University of London

Dr Jonathan Mann   World Health Organisation, Geneva

Professor A A Glynn   Head, PHLS AIDS Centre

Professor N J Bailey   Hôpital Cantonal Universitaire, Geneva

Dr Joan Aron   John Hopkins School of Public Health

Dr T Peterman   Centers for Disease Control
AIDS Unit, Atlanta

Dr N S Galbraith   Director, PHLS Communicable
Diseases Surveillance Centre

Dr D B L McClelland   Blood Transfusion Service Scotland

Dr M McEvoy   PHLS Communicable Diseases
Surveillance Centre

Professor M J R Healy   London School of Hygiene and
Tropical Medicine

Dr H Tillett   PHLS Communicable Diseases
Surveillance Centre

Dr Dan Reid   Communicable Diseases (Scotland) Unit

Professor M Alder   Middlesex Hospital, London

Dr Philip Mortimer   PHLS Virus Reference Laboratory,
Colindale

Scientific Observers:

Dr Anne Johnson	Middlesex Hospital, London
Dr Johan Giesecke	Karolinska Hospital, Stockholm
Professor Hekker	State Institute for Health and Hygiene, Netherlands

Government Observers:

Mr Anthony Langdon	Cabinet Office
Professor Keith McAdam	Social Services Committee
Mr C D Daykin	Government Actuary's Department
Ms Jacqui Mallinder	Treasury
Dr R Covell	Scottish Home & Health Department
Mr T S Heppell	Department of Health & Social Security
Dr E Harris	Department of Health & Social Security
Dr H Pickles	Department of Health & Social Security
Dr Richard Gibbs	Department of Health & Social Security
Dr G Greenberg	Department of Health & Social Security
Mr A B Barton	Department of Health & Social Security
Mr Robert Anderson	Department of Health & Social Security

Secretariat:

Dr Fenton Lewis	Department of Health & Social Security
Mrs M Beeston	Department of Health & Social Security

Printed in the United Kingdom for Her Majesty's Stationery Office.
Dd.289948, 12/87, C20, 434, 5673.